The M
Syndrome
in Clinical Practice

WA 12962

D1765023

The Metabolic Syndrome in Clinical Practice

Satish Mittal

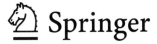 Springer

Satish Mittal, MBBS
General Medical Practitioner
Esher
UK

(formerly, General Practice Principal, East Molesey, East Surrey
Health Authority, Surrey, UK; and Clinical Governance Lead cum
Chairman Clinical Governance Committee, East Elmbridge
Primary Care Group, Esher, Surrey, UK; formerly, Medical
Registrar, Southlands Hospital, Shoreham-by Sea, and Registrar
in Cardiology at Preston Hall Hospital, Maidstone, Kent, UK.)

Cover photograph by Dr. Satish Mittal

British Library Cataloguing in Publication Data

Mittal, Satish
   The metabolic syndrome in clinical practice
   1. Metabolic syndrome
   I. Title
   616.3'9

Library of Congress Control Number: 2008929187

ISBN 978-1-84628-910-1   e-ISBN 978-1-84628-911-8

© Springer-Verlag London Limited 2008

Apart from any fair dealing for the purposes of research or private study, or
criticism or review, as permitted under the Copyright, Designs and Patents
Act 1988, this publication may only be reproduced, stored or transmitted, in
any form or by any means, with the prior permission in writing of the publishers, or in the case of reprographic reproduction in accordance with the
terms of licences issued by the Copyright Licensing Agency. Enquiries concerning reproduction outside those terms should be sent to the publishers.

The use of registered names, trademarks, etc. in this publication does not
imply, even in the absence of a specific statement, that such names are exempt
from the relevant laws and regulations and therefore free for general use.

Product liability: The publisher can give no guarantee for information
about drug dosage and application thereof contained in this book. In every
individual case the respective user must check its accuracy by consulting
other pharmaceutical literature.

9 8 7 6 5 4 3 2 1

Springer Science + Business Media

springer.com

Learning Resources
Centre

12962473

Dedicated to my sons Vijay, Ashok, Ajay and
in memory of my parents Harish Chandra
and Ramanandi

Preface

This book addresses the current issues about, and treatments for, the metabolic syndrome and its components, specifically obesity, diabetes, and cardiovascular disease. Cross-sectional surveys indicate that one third of adults and an alarming proportion of children in the United States have the metabolic syndrome, which also represents a global public health problem.

In 1988 Gerald Reaven first delivered his Banting lecture, "The Role of Insulin Resistance in Human Disease," and the following year Harold Himsworth delivered the Goulstonian lecture, "Mechanisms of Diabetes," to the Royal College of Physicians in London. Since then, an abundance of research has been conducted in the pathophysiology, epidemiology, and therapeutic strategies of the metabolic syndrome. Yet today there is no other topic in medicine that has provoked as much discussion as this syndrome; its precise cause has been debated, and even its very existence and usefulness has been challenged. These issues are addressed with sensitivity in this book. Whether it is called the metabolic syndrome (Scott Grundy), the insulin resistance syndrome (Reaven), or an "emperor without clothes" (Richard Kahn), it appears to be a simple syndrome in its clinical approach but it still remains a defiant problem.

This book serves as a resource on this topic for primary care physicians, medical students, residents in internal medicine, nurse practitioners, and those who wish to update and improve their knowledge in the field of the newly emerging science of the metabolic syndrome.

This book provides a practical and sensible approach to the understanding of insulin resistance and obesity/hypertriglyceridemic waist as underlying incriminating factors in the causation of the metabolic syndrome. It is written in a question-and-answer format, and the questions are carefully selected to address the issues relevant to clinical practice, for which it is thoroughly referenced. The components of the metabolic syndrome are dealt with in depth, which is crucial for understanding this syndrome. The book includes chapters on components of the metabolic syndrome, pathophysiology, outcome, diagnostic criteria, and clinical implications. The components that form the basis of the syndrome are dealt with in detail, including insulin resistance, obesity, adipokines, dyslipidemia, proinflammatory and prothrombotic states, hypertension, and glucose intolerance, among others. The pathogenesis of the syndrome includes the role of fatty acids and other incriminating factors. Recent evidence regarding outcome is presented as it relates the metabolic syndrome to cardiovascular disease (CVD), diabetes, fatty liver, polycystic ovary syndrome (PCOS), and sleep apnea. The diagnostic criteria are displayed in tables. The chapter on clinical implications provides up-to-date referenced evidence for lifestyle modification and the pharmacological role in the management of metabolic syndrome, and consequently the reduction of cardiovascular disease and diabetes. Readers should consult the medication's prescribing information and guidelines relevant to their national formulary.

I am thankful to my wife, Zulaika, for typing the script despite her own heavy schedule at home and at work, and to my sons, Ajay and Ashok, for contributing the tables and illustrations.

Contents

Chapter 1
Introduction

PREVALENCE

Q: What factors affect the prevalence of the metabolic syndrome and its variations among different populations?

The concept of the metabolic syndrome has existed for at least 80 years. In 1920, Kylin, a Swedish physician, first described a constellation of metabolic disturbance, which entailed the risk factors of cardiovascular disease (CVD), atherosclerotic cardiovascular disease (ASCVD), and the clustering of hypertension, hyperglycemia, and gout [1]. In 1988, Reaven [2] postulated that several risk factors—dyslipidemia, hyperglycemia, and hypertension—commonly cluster together, which he recognized as the multiple risk factors for CVD, which he called syndrome X. Reaven and subsequently others postulated that insulin resistance underlines syndrome X; therefore, another commonly used term was *insulin resistance syndrome*. The concept of this syndrome was based on the resistance to metabolic actions of insulin. Therefore, hyperinsulinemia, glucose intolerance, type 2 diabetes, hypertriglyceridemia, and low high-density lipoprotein (HDL) cholesterol concentration can be explained due to resistance to the action of insulin on carbohydrate and lipid metabolism. However, the National Cholesterol Education Program's (NCEP) Adult Treatment Panel (ATP-III) prefers the term *metabolic syndrome* as it avoids implicating insulin resistance as the only or primary cause of this syndrome. The concept of the metabolic syndrome has been accepted by most international authorities, but controversies still exist about its cause. There is a consensus on the essential components of metabolic syndrome—obesity, glucose intolerance, hypertension, and dyslipidemia—but opinions differ on other components. In 1998, an initiative was set up to develop an internationally agreed upon definition of the metabolic syndrome. (This is discussed in a later chapter.)

The metabolic syndrome is also referred to by various other names, such as deadly quartet, metabolic cardiovascular risk syndrome, and dysmetabolic syndrome, among others.

The unadjusted prevalence of the metabolic syndrome increased from 23.1% in the National Health and Nutrition Examination Survey (NHANES-III) to 26.7% in NHANES 1999–2000. The age-adjusted prevalence of the metabolic syndrome increased from 24.1% in NHANES-III to 27% in NHANES 1999–2000. Among women, the unadjusted prevalence increased by a relative 25.8%. Corresponding increases among men were very small and were not statistically significant. Among women increases occurred among all age groups, and the increases among women aged 20 to 39 years was significant. Among men, nonsignificant increases occurred among participants aged 20 to 39 and 40 to 59 years [3].

The association of the metabolic syndrome with diabetes is highlighted by NHANES-III analysis, which found that approximately 85% of individuals with diabetes had metabolic syndrome as compared to only 12% of those who had normal fasting glucose [4]. Most studies undertaken in developed countries and urban areas of developing countries suggest a prevalence of 15% to 20% of the general adult population based on NCEP ATP-III criteria. Moreover, if the International Diabetic Federation (IDF) definition is applied, the prevalence will be greater. The prevalence was similar or higher using World Health Organization (WHO) criteria as compared to NCEP ATP-III criteria, but for Mexican men and women the reverse was true. Using the impaired glucose tolerance (IGT) test in ATP-III criteria increased the prevalence by 5%. The factors that affect the prevalence of the metabolic syndrome are modifiable or nonmodifiable and are interlinked.

Despite the attempts in recent years to agree on a universally acceptable definition of the metabolic syndrome, it remains difficult to compare the prevalence in various populations as the published data differ with regard to their study design, sample selection, the year of the study, the definition used for the metabolic syndrome, and the age and sex of the study population. Reviewing various studies that include a population sample aged 20 to 25 years and older, the prevalence in urban populations varies from 8% (India) to 24% (United States) in men and from 7% (France) to 46% (India) in women [5] (Table 1.1). Interestingly, of the three studies listed in the table, two Indian studies differed in their definition of obesity. Ramachandran et al [6] from Chennai, India, used a waist circumference that is appropriate

TABLE 1.1. Prevalence of metabolic syndrome in worldwide populations

Country or town	Age	Gender M	F	Criteria	Reference
Jaipur	>20	7.9	17.5	ATP-III	[7]
Chennai	>20	36.4	46.5	ATP-III	[6]
Chennai	20–75	12.9	9.9	EGIR	[8]
Australia	>55	19.5	17.2	ATP-III	N.A.**
England	40–65	44.8	30.90	WHO	[30]
France	30–65	23.5	9.6	WHO	[30]
Italy	40–81	34.5	18.0	WHO	[30]
Iran	>20	24	42	ATP-III	[10]
Mexico	20–69	26.6	*	ATP-III	[31]
Holland	20–60	19.9	7.6	WHO	[30]
Spain	30–64	25.5	19.9	WHO	[30]
Sweden	46–68	43.3	26.3	WHO	[30]
U.S.	30–79	24.7	21.3	ATP-III	[18]
U.S.	30–79	29.0	32.8	ATP-III	[18]

ATP-III, Adult Treatment Panel; WHO, World Health Organization.
*N.A.
Source: Cameron et al [5].
**Data from the International Diabetic Institute Melbourne 2003.

for Indians, while Gupta et al [7] used the standard ATP-III definition of obesity. Both studies were similar in using population-based samples within the same age range, but the prevalence was 13% in Jaipur, India, as reported by Gupta and 41% in Chennai, India as reported by Ramachandran. Despite this disparity, it is interesting to note that the prevalence of obesity in the two study groups was quite similar (31% vs. 33%). However, much larger differences were observed between the two studies for the prevalence of elevated triglycerides (46% vs. 30%), hypertension (55% vs. 39%), and elevated fasting plasma glucose (25% vs. 5%), each of which had used the same cutoff point—the ATP definition. A third study from Chennai by Deepa et al [8], however, reported a prevalence of 11.2% using European Group for the study of Insulin Resistance (EGIR) criteria; the results of this study were similar to those of the study in Jaipur. Therefore, even within the same ethnic population group it appears that there can be significant differences in the prevalence of both the individual factors that constitute the metabolic syndrome and the metabolic syndrome itself [5]. The prevalence of the metabolic syndrome also depends on its components (Table 1.2) [9].

TABLE 1.2. Prevalence of metabolic syndrome and its components

Components	Men		Women	
	45–54	55–64	45–54	55–64
Metabolic syndrome	36.2	41.4	16.5	27.9
NGT with IR	12.2	9.5	15.1	15.0
Impaired fasting glucose	14.5	12.4	5.8	3.6
Impaired glucose tolerance	8.9	13.8	6.9	12.6
Diabetes	7.5	12.6	5.2	8.3
Obesity	77.6	81.9	26.9	39.4

IR, insulin resistance; NGT, normal glucose tolerance.
Source: Llannie-Parikka et al [9].

Age

The prevalence of the metabolic syndrome increases with age. On the basis of the 2002 census, approximately 47 million U.S. residents have the metabolic syndrome [3]. The unadjusted and age-adjusted prevalence of the metabolic syndrome for adults were 21.8 and 23.7%, respectively. The prevalence increased from 6.7% among people aged 20 through 29 years to 43.5% and 42.0% for participants aged 60 through 69 years and aged 70 years and older, respectively. Mexican Americans had the highest age-adjusted prevalence of metabolic syndrome (31.0%). The age-adjusted prevalence is similar for men (24%) and women (23.4%). However, among African Americans, women had about a 57% higher prevalence than did men, and Mexican American women had a 26% higher prevalence than did men. The prevalence of two or more components of the metabolic syndrome is 43.9%, showing that a large group is at risk of its development. The prevalence in Iran is less than 10% for both men and women in the 20- to 29-year age group, rising to 38% and 67%, respectively, in the 60- to 69-year age group [10]. Likewise, in the French population, the prevalence rises from <5.6% in the 30- to 39-year age group to 17.5% in the 60- to 64-year age group [10].

Gender

There is wide variation in the prevalence in men and women. Prevalence is high in Europeans men, as they tend to be more obese [11]. However, in populations where women are more obese, their prevalence correspondingly increases. The association of metabolic disorders with the metabolic syndrome is different in men and women [12]. The French study suggested that elevated body weight and waist girth and low HDL cholesterol are significantly larger contributors to the metabolic syndrome in women than in men;

regulation of glucose and lipid metabolism. Insulin is essential for the appropriate development, growth, and maintenance of whole-body glucose homeostasis. This hormone is secreted by the β cells of the pancreatic islets of Langerhans in response to increased circulatory levels of glucose and amino acids after meal. Insulin secretion is matched by circulating glucose level. Insulin is secreted at regular pulses at a low basal level (this is responsible for 50% of daily secretion) and in close temporal association to the rise in portal plasma glucose after meals. Blood levels are closely regulated in health and rarely go outside the range of 3.5 to 8 mmol/L (63 to 144 mg/dL), despite the varying demand of food, during fasting, postprandially, and during exercise. Small amounts of basal insulin are continuously released, and these levels are exquisitely sensitive to changes in the blood glucose level.

Being a pleiotropic hormone, insulin has a range of actions such as glucoregulation and antilipolysis and protein synthesis. The action of insulin depends on the level of circulating insulin and the shape of the individual's insulin dose-response curve. After secretion, insulin enters the portal circulation and is carried to the liver, the prime target organ. Approximately half of secreted insulin is extracted and degraded in the liver; the residue is broken down by the kidneys. Insulin plays a central integrating role during fasting and feeding states. In the fasting state, when the insulin concentration is low, insulin mainly acts as hepatic hormone, modulating glucose production (via glycogenolysis and gluconeogenesis) from the liver. However, in the postprandial state when insulin concentration is high, it suppresses glucose production from the liver and promotes the entry of glucose into the peripheral tissues (i.e. fat, muscles) and increases glucose utilization. Insulin plays a role in lowering blood glucose in the following ways: (1) suppression of hepatic glucose output (via decreased gluconeogenesis and glycogenolysis) and thus reducing the rate of circulatory glucose supply; and (2) stimulation of glucose disposal, primarily into striated muscle and adipose tissue. In the muscle and fat cells, the clearance of circulating glucose depends on the insulin-stimulated translocation of the glucose transporter GLUT-4 isoform of the cell surface. Normal actions of insulin are summarized in Table 1.3.

Hepatic Glucose Production

Hepatic glucose production is the main determinant of fasting blood glucose concentration. In the postabsorptive state (i.e., after an 8- to 12-hour overnight fast), the liver controls the rate at which glucose enters the circulation; the initial source of glucose is due to breakdown of stored glycogen. But as hepatic stores get

TABLE 1.3. Actions of insulin

Conventional biological effects

Muscle	↑ Glucose uptake and utilization, ↑ glycogenosis, ↓ lipolysis, ↓ glycogenolysis, ↓ glyconeogenesis, ↓ amino acids, ↓ protein catabolism
Hepatic	↑ Glycogen synthesis, ↓ glycogenolysis, ↓ gluconeogenesis, VLDL secretion
Kidneys	↑ Sodium retention, ↑ uric acid clearance, ↓ gluconeogenesis
Fat	↑ Lipoprotein lipase activity, ↑ uptake of circulatory fat & utilization, ↑ glucose uptake and utilization
Circulation	↓ Uric acid formation, ↑ NO synthesis

Novel biological effects

Antiinflammatory	↓ NF-κB, ↑ I-κB, ↓ MCP, ↓ ICAM, ↓ CRP
Antioxidant	↓ ROS
Antithrombotic	↓ TF
Prothrombotic	↓ PAI-1
Antiatherosclerotic	ApoE null mouse, IRS-1 and -2 null mouse
Platelet inhibition	↑ NO release in platelets, ↑ cAMP
Vasodilatory	↑ NO release, ↑ eNOS expression
Antiapoptotic	Heart, lungs, etc.

cAMP, cyclic adenosine monophosphate; CRP, C-reactive protein; eNOS, endothelial nitric oxide synthase; ICAM, intercellular adhesion molecule; IRS, insulin receptor substrate; MCP, monocyte chemotactic protein; NF-κB, nuclear factor κB; NO, nitric oxide; PAI, plasminogen activator inhibitor; ROS, reactive oxygen species; TF, tissue factor; VLDL, very low density lipoprotein.

depleted, usually after 24 hours, liver synthesizes de novo glucose. The principal action of insulin is to suppress glucose production, and the development of type 2 diabetes is the result mainly of inadequate suppression of this gluconeogenesis.

Glucose Disposal

Stimulation of glucose disposal by skeletal muscles requires higher insulin level than the one required for suppression of hepatic gluconeogenesis. The stimulation of intracellular translocation of GLUT-4 glucose transporters to the cell membrane is the key role of insulin to fulfill this function of glucose disposal. GLUT-4 is profusely expressed in skeletal and heart muscle, and also in adipose tissue. Other isoforms of glucose transporters do not need insulin for translocation to the cell membrane.

Lipolysis and Ketone Body

Insulin also profoundly affects lipid metabolism, increasing lipid synthesis in liver and fat cells, and decreasing fatty acids release from triglycerides in fat and muscle. Insulin also modulates transcription, altering the cell content of numerous messenger RNAs (mRNAs). It stimulates growth, DNA synthesis, and cell replication. Insulin is also secreted in response to other secretagogues such as amino acids but its secretion is inhibited by adrenaline, epinephrine, and somatostatin. Its secretion is increased by glucagon and gastric-inhibiting polypeptide.

Q: What are the novel biological effects of insulin?

The tight control of glucose concentration is determined by a balance between glucose absorption from the intestine, glucose production by the liver, and glucose uptake from the plasma. In tissues, such as fat, muscle, and liver, glucose uptake or storage is regulated by insulin, but insulin has no significant role to play in stimulating glucose metabolism in the brain, kidney, and erythrocytes. Insulin also plays an anabolic role promoting the storage of substrate in fat, liver, and muscles by stimulating lipogenesis and glycogen and protein synthesis, inhibiting lipolysis, glycogenolysis, and protein breakdown; and stimulating cell growth and differentiation.

Insulin resistance in individuals with type 2 diabetes is defined by defects in insulin-stimulated glucose transport, glycogen synthesis, and glucose oxidation, but other pathways may also be altered. Up to 75% of insulin-dependent glucose disposal occurs in skeletal muscle, whereas adipose tissue accounts for only 5% to 15%. Adipose tissue also exerts its role in glucose homeostasis through its release of free fatty acids (FFAs), tumor necrosis factor-α (TNF-α), leptin, Acrp 30/adiponectin, and other adipokines that have been shown to contribute to insulin action and insulin resistance. Treatment of type 2 diabetes with insulin for 2 weeks reduces C-reactive protein (CRP) and monocyte chemotactic protein-1 (MCP-1) [19]. Treatment with insulin results in a rapid marked decrease in the concentration of inflammatory mediators in patients with severe hyperglycemia associated with markedly increases in inflammatory markers. Insulin was also shown to reduce inflammatory mediators (i.e., interleukin-1β [IL-1β], IL-6, macrophage migration inhibitor factor [MIF], TNF-α), and expression of proinflammatory transcription factors CEBP (C enhancer binding protein) and cytokines in the liver in experimental animals [19].

Insulin suppresses AP-1 activating protein and Egr-1 (early response growth factor-1), two proinflammatory transcription factors and their respective genes, matrix metalloproteinase-9 (MMP-9), tissue factor (TF), and plasminogen activator inhibitor-1 (PAI-1). Thus, insulin has both an antiinflammatory and antioxidant effect as supported by its ability to suppress reactive oxygen species (ROS) generation and p47^{phos} expression. Egr-1 is the transcription factor that modulates TF, which in turn activates thrombin generation. Insulin increases I-κB (inhibitor-κB) expression in mononuclear cells (MNCs) as well as suppresses plasma concentration of intercellular adhesion molecule-1 and monocyte chemotactic protein-1 [19]. Insulin also has an antioxidant effect as shown by its ability to suppress ROS generation and p47^{phox} expression. The effects of insulin indicate that insulin could have a crucial inhibitory role in the regulation of factors that are central to atherogenesis, plaque rupture, and thrombosis (Fig. 1.1).

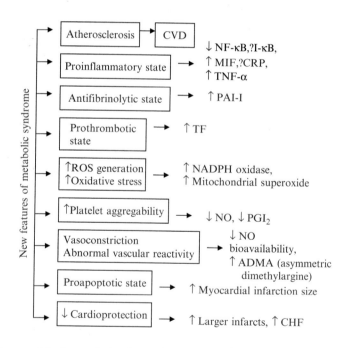

FIGURE 1.1. Interrelationship of metabolic syndrome and its novel actions of insulin. ADMA (asymmetric dimethylargine), CHF, congestive heart failure; CRP, C-reactive protein; CVD, cardiovascular disease; MIF, migration inhibitor factor; NADPH, reduced nicotinamide adenine dinucleotide phosphate; NF, nuclear factor; NO, nitric oxide; PAI, plasminogen activator inhibitor; PGI$_2$, prostaglandin I$_2$; TF, tissue factor TNF-α, tumor necrosis factor-α. (From Dandona et al [19].)

Insulin also has an antiapoptotic effect. It is supported by experimental studies in animals [19] in which the addition of insulin to the reperfusion fluid led to a reduction in myocardial infarction size by 50% [19]. In a human study, infusion of insulin at a low dose with a heparin and thrombolytic agent produced a cardioprotective effect. Additionally, patients with the insulin resistance state of obesity and type 2 diabetes suffered larger myocardial infarcts as compared to nondiabetics [19]. Insulin administration suppresses atherogenesis in the apolipoprotein E (ApoE)-null mouse [19]. Conversely, interference with insulin signal transduction, as in the insulin receptor substrate-2 (IRS-2) null mouse, results in atherosclerosis. The IRS-1 null mouse also had a tendency toward atherosclerosis. It is noticed that a mutation of IRS-1 (arginine-792) causes abnormal vascular reactivity, a decrease in endothelial nitric oxide synthase (eNOS) expression in endothelial cells, and an increased incidence of CHD. Insulin sensitizers such as rosiglitazone have been shown to have an antiinflammatory effect in addition to their glucose lowering effect in diabetics. Metformin causes a reduction in the plasma concentration of MIF in the obese [20].

Q: How does the signaling mechanism that regulates glucose transport work?

The intracellular insulin-signaling cascade plays an important role in insulin action and in the development of insulin resistance. There are two major postreceptor signaling pathways that convey the insulin signaling downstream. One pathway, involving the phosphorylation of IRS-1 and -2 and activation of phosphatidylinositol (PI)-3-kinase, which appears to be absolutely necessary for mediating the metabolic effects of insulin. The second signaling pathway appears to involve the phosphorylation of Shc and activation of Ras, Raf, MEK, and mitogen-activated protein (MAP) kinase (Erk-1 and -2). In contrast to the IRS/PI-3-kinase pathway, activation of the Shc-Ras MAP kinase intermediates contributes solely to the nucleus and mitogenic effects of insulin and plays no role in conveying the metabolic action of insulin. In individuals who develop insulin resistance, the impaired insulin action leads to activation of proinflammatory transcription factor and an increase in the expression of corresponding genes.

Insulin Action and Insulin Receptor

Insulin action is initiated through the binding to and activation of its cell-surface receptor. The insulin receptor is a large transmembrane glycoprotein of about 350 kDa, composed of α and β subunits. Insulin binds the extracellular and subunits, transmitting a signal across the plasma membrane that activates the intracellular tyrosine kinase domain of the β subunit. Translation of the mRNA yields a proreceptor that is glycosylated and forms disulfide links before cleavage to form the mature receptor. This inserts into the plasma membrane. The cytosol of β subunits carries protein tyrosine kinase, which like other receptors can phosphorylate within the cytosolic domain of the receptor, a process known as autophosphorylation. This process is initiated when the receptor is activated by binding insulin. Also, the tyrosine kinase activity can phosphorylate tyrosines in target proteins, two of which are IRS-1 and -2. This results in binding and activating other signaling proteins, one of the most important of which is PI-3-kinase.

Tyrosine kinase activity of the insulin receptor decreases as a result of serine/threonine phosphorylation. Hyperinsulinemia associated with insulin resistance might stimulate the relevant serine kinase, perhaps through the insulin-like growth factor (IGF-1) receptor, which can also be stimulated by elevated insulin levels. Such an interaction could provide a mechanism for a vicious cycle of insulin-induced insulin resistance. Likewise, counterregulatory hormones and cytokines can activate serine kinases, particularly protein kinase C (PKC), which is implicated in the development of peripheral insulin resistance.

Pharmacological inhibition of PKC activity or reduction of PKC expression increases insulin sensitivity and insulin receptor tyrosine kinase activity [21]. Several protein tyrosine phosphatases (PTPases) (e.g., PTPIB and LAR) have been implicated that can dephosphorylate the insulin receptor, reducing its kinase activity, and subsequently reducing insulin action. This finding is supported by the evidence that each of these phosphates is elevated in insulin-resistant individuals [21]. There is no single or common defect that underlines the peripheral insulin resistance. It is a complex phenomenon in which several genetic defects combine with environmental stresses, such as obesity, or infections, to generate the phenotype.

In addition to tyrosine phosphorylation, the insulin receptor is also subjected to β subunit serine/threonine phosphorylation; this modification allows the receptor function to be attenuated [22]. Various pathways of phosphorylation and dephosphorylation reactions leading from these substrates result in the activation or suppression of insulin-sensitive enzymes such as activation of glycogen synthase, which converts glucose-6-phosphate to glycogen. The other pathways produce genomic effects of insulin—the repression of phosphoenolpyruvate carboxykinase (PEPCK), for example, an important enzyme in the pathway of gluconeogenesis that converts oxaloacetate to phosphoenolpyruvate. Glucose uptake via the GLUT-4 isoform of mammalian hexose transporters accounts for most of the stimulatory effect of insulin on this process in muscle and fat cells. GLUT-4 rapidly recycles through the plasma membrane/endosomal membrane system in the presence of insulin [23]. In the case of the insulin receptor, tyrosine phosphorylation of four related substrates (IRS) proteins and Gab-1 causes many candidate signaling proteins to be recruited, including the following:

1. The p110-type PI-3-kinase
2. Grb-2 and protein tyrosine phosphatase SH-PTP-2, which seems essential for p21^{ras} activation [23], and tyrosine kinase Fyn, which in turn activates PI-3-kinase and p21^{ras} pathways
3. Rho-associated protein serine/threonine kinase ROKα [23]

PI-3-kinase activity is clearly necessary for insulin-stimulated glucose uptake. Insulin receptor signaling can also involve p21^{ras} through tyrosine phosphorylation of Shc and its subsequent binding to complexes of Grb2 and Sos. p21^{ras} and PI-3-kinase are two important initial switch elements for insulin signaling. There is involvement of multiple protein serine/threonine kinases downstream of both the p21^{ras} and PI-3-kinase elements. Two classes of serine/threonine kinases are known to act downstream of PI-3-kinase, namely the serine/threonine kinase Akt, also known as protein kinase B (PKB) and the atypical PKC isoforms ζ (zeta) and λ (lambda). Expression of PKC ζ and λ are also observed to induce GLUT-4 translocation, whereas expression of a dominant-interfering PKC λ inhibited GLUT-4 translocation [12].

Another recently discovered class of likely downstream effectors of 3-phosphoinositides include proteins that regulate membrane-related functions, such as actin assembly (Rac guanosine triphosphatase [GTPase]), early endosome fusion (EEAI), and guanine nucleotide exchange (GRP1 [general receptor for phosphoinositidesi], cytohesin-1, and ARNO [ARF-nucleotide-binding site opener]) or possibly GTPase activation (α-centaurin) of ARF [ADP-ribosylation factor] proteins (Fig. 1.2) [23]. With further research, more and more downstream effectors of insulin signaling are likely to be added. From the constant efforts to find which of the above insulin receptor signaling elements is actually linked to GLUT-4 translocation, there is strong support for PI-3-kinase activity rather than p21^{ras} function. However, there are potential gaps in our present knowledge. Another cell signaling pathway that seems to markedly stimulate glucose uptake in muscle involves nitric oxide (NO). In the recent years, new

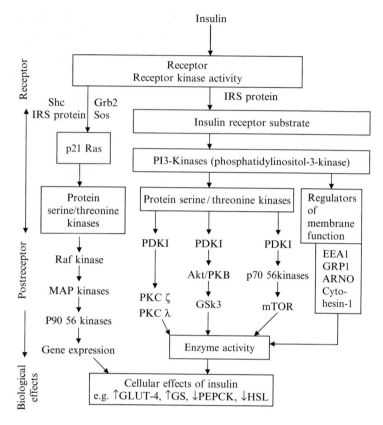

FIGURE 1.2. Pathways of insulin signaling. GLUT, glucose transporter; GS, glycogen synthase; HSL, hormone-sensitive lipase; IRS, insulin receptor substrate; MAP, mitogen-activated protein; PDK, phosphoinositide-dependent kinase; PEPCK, phosphoenolpyruvate carboxykinase; PI, phosphatidylinositol; PKB, protein kinase B; Ras, rat sarcoma protein. (From Czech and Corvera [23].)

components of the insulin receptor signaling network have been discovered and their complementary DNA (cDNA) clones isolated [23].

Recently discovered downstream targets of insulin-regulated PI-3-kinase lipid products, including protein kinase C isoforms λ and ζ, regulatory protein kinase of the Akt/protein kinase B system, tyrosine kinases 1tk/Btk/Tec, the early endosome regulator EEA1, and ARF exchange factors, GRP1 general receptor for phosphoinositides 1, ARNO, and cytohesin-1. It is also possible that newly discovered additional cellular signaling elements such as trimeric G protein, NO, and cyclic guanosine monophosphate (cGMP) can regulate glucose transport and that unknown signaling events may be needed in addition to PI-3-kinase for insulin action [23].

Q: What are the levels of impaired insulin action?
There are four different arbitrarily sites of action: prereceptor, receptor, postreceptor, or effector defects. In the majority, the effects are a combination of both genetic and environmental factors. Genetic causes include altered expression levels of genes including receptors, transporters, signaling intermediates, and metabolic enzymes responsible for insulin signaling and nutrient metabolism. Environmental factors include nutrients, cytokines, hormones, and drugs.

Prereceptor/Receptor Defects
Prereceptor defects include reduced insulin availability, insulin antibodies, and structurally defective insulin. They do not contribute significantly in the development of type 2 diabetes. Receptor defects include a reduced number of receptors or a reduced receptor affinity for insulin. This may occur in response to chronic hyperinsulinism (so-called downregulation). Reduced insulin receptor binding associated with obesity or glucose intolerance is reversible by treatment [22].

Postreceptor defects refer to intracellular events occurring after insulin has bound to its receptor. This appears to be the major cause of insulin resistance in type 2 diabetes and is only partially amenable to treatment. The precise method of these intracellular events are not elucidated, but reduction in the insulin-stimulated tyrosine phosphorylation of IRS-1 and decreased activity of the subsequent signaling intermediates such as PI-3-kinase and protein kinase B have been observed in individuals with type 2 diabetes. It is likely that insulin insensitivity in obesity and type 2 diabetes is the result of a cumulative effect of various small changes in the degree of expression and activities of these intermediates. Some forms of insulin resistance may be due to the receptor itself. Alterations in insulin receptor expression, binding, phosphorylation state, or kinase activity may be responsible for several insulin-resistance phenotypes. It is likely that selected blockage of distinct phosphorylation sites selectively inhibits certain actions of insulin. For example, some individuals have been observed to have rare genetic defects in the insulin receptor that affect expression, ligand binding, and tyrosine kinase activity. These individuals manifest severe insulin resistance clinically as different syndromes including the type A syndrome, leprechaunism, Rabson-Mendenhall syndrome, and lipoatrophic diabetes.

The mode of inheritance found in affected families with insulin receptor mutations provides some knowledge about insulin receptor function. Most people with severe familial insulin resistance carry lesions in both insulin receptor (INSR) alleles, either as homozygotes or compound heterozygotes. In these patients the whole cellular complement of the insulin receptor is defective [21]. However, some cases of type A syndrome of insulin resistance (characterized by polycystic ovarian disease, signs of virilization, acanthosis nigricans, and enhanced growth rate) affected individuals with apparently simple heterozygotes and only one defective allele [21].

Effector Defects

As the term implies, *effector defects* refer to the disturbances or impairment in the final products of the insulin signaling pathways such as events involving glucose transporters and glucoregulatory enzymes. The insulin-stimulated translocation for the main insulin-sensitive glucose transporter (GLUT-4) to the plasma membrane of the muscle cell is impaired in type 2 diabetes, whereas the transporters themselves remain structurally normal, as are the insulin-sensitive enzymes [22]. This is indicative of incrimination of insulin-signaling pathways governing the translocation of glucose transporters to the plasma membrane, and the activities of important glucoregulatory enzymes are the main sites of defective function responsible for insulin resistance.

Furthermore, persistent hyperglycemia and dyslipidemia may cause insulin resistance by damaging mitochondrial function, which in turn increases ROS within cells, and the oxidative stress impairs insulin signaling, glucose, and lipid metabolism. Finally, the insulin action at the tissue level may be antagonized by counterregulatory hormones such as glucagon, catecholamines, glucocorticoids, and growth hormone. These hormones act directly on insulin signaling, glucose transporters, and glucoregulatory enzymes in target tissues.

THE THRIFTY GENO- AND PHENOTYPE HYPOTHESIS

Q: What is the link among the thrifty geno- and phenotype hypothesis, low birth weight, and the metabolic syndrome?

There is a relationship of low birth weight with hypertension, visceral obesity, dyslipidemia, a prothrombotic state, and CHD. It is postulated that fetal malnutrition predisposes to the metabolic syndrome; the exact mechanism, however, is unclear. Several studies have shown that blood pressure, type 2 diabetes, or insulin resistance, or a combination of them, is consistently related to low birth weight. There is some evidence that low birth weight has some association with insulin resistance syndrome, probably due to environmental factors. Low birth weight is associated with higher prevalence of the metabolic syndrome in adult life [24]. Furthermore, the effect of low birth weight on increased risk for the metabolic syndrome appears to be particularly greater when it is associated with obesity in adulthood [25].

In 1962, Neel [26] proposed the thrifty genotype hypothesis, aiming to address the etiology of diabetes. He proposes that the predisposition to diabetes might arise because of genetic variations that were advantageous in certain environmental situations but were later made injurious in a different environment. He suggested that the different prevalences of type 2 diabetes and the different genetic predispositions to diabetes are the result of different forces of selection due to nutritional circumstances in various populations. This is in contrast to the thrifty phenotype hypothesis, which suggests early environmental influence acting to increase the risk of type 2 diabetes. Neel suggested the thrifty genotype hypothesis, in which the emergence of insulin resistance and diabetes in populations shifting from vigorous activity and subsistence nutrition to abundance and obesity of urban societies. Neel hypothesized that certain populations have a higher prevalence of genetic traits that once offered survival advantages during protracted periods of meager nutrient supply, but that may be injurious due to abundant food supplies and reduced habitual physical activity.

Hales and Barker in 1992 proposed the basis of the thrifty phenotype hypothesis [32]. They hypothesized that the epidemiological associations between poor fetal and infant growth and the subsequent development of type 2 diabetes and the metabolic syndrome result from the effects of poor nutrition in early life, which produces permanent changes in glucose-insulin metabolism. These changes include reduced capacity for insulin secretion and insulin resistance, which, together with the effects of obesity, aging, and physical inactivity, are crucial determinants in the development of type 2 diabetes

Hale and Barker suggest that in response to poor fetal nutrition the compromised fetus adopts a number of defensive measures to increase its chances of survival. These strategies include growth of the brain, which is spared at the expense of other tissues (such as muscles, kidneys, and the endocrine pancreas), and metabolic programming is adopted to the conditions akin to poor postnatal nutrition. For instance, the fetus adapts by storing nutrients such as fat. Once this fetal programming takes place, the problem does not arise so long as the fetus is born in an environment of poor nutritional status. However, if birth takes place in conditions of adequate or overnutrition, this situation conflicts with the in-utero programming and it results in obesity, type 2 diabetes, and other features of the metabolic syndrome. Such situations arise when the population that migrated from poor areas with undernutrition to areas with adequate or overnutrition (e.g., Western areas). This theory provides an alternative to the previous concept of the thrifty genotype hypothesis. It proposes that type 2 diabetes results, at least in part, from relative intrauterine malnutrition and that the latter leads to lifelong metabolic programming, which includes a reduced complement of islet β cells combined with insulin resistance in skeletal muscle. There is substantial evidence to show a correlation between low birth weight and an increased risk of type 2 diabetes in middle age. The other cardiovascular risk factors, such as hypertension, have also been linked to low birth weight.

This concept is applicable to several ethnic populations including South Indians. The consensus of opinion is that across many ethnic populations there is a consistent association between birth weight and insulin resistance later in life. Interestingly, if individuals of low socioeconomic status who were born small remain small, without rapid weight gain or a catch up in growth in childhood, then the risk of insulin resistance remains [27]. Low birth weight also may be due to environmental factors. It has been shown that low birth weight and other measures of small size at birth can also be associated with a higher level of several cardiovascular disease risk factors. Infants of low birth weight have been noted to have elevated levels of the components of insulin resistance syndrome in adult life. They have high blood pressure, as well as elevated plasma glucose, insulin levels (both fasting and after a standard oral glucose load), and plasma triglycerides. They also have low HDL cholesterol, but low-density lipoprotein (LDL) cholesterol is not affected. The offspring of women with a low BMI in pregnancy had elevated 3-hour plasma insulin levels in adulthood, which indicates that they were insulin resistant. They also had reduced glucose tolerance.

Phillip and colleagues [28] have shown that fasting plasma cortisol concentration in men is inversely correlated with birth weight and positively correlated with systolic blood pressure, fasting and 2-hour plasma glucose level during an oral glucose tolerance test, plasma triglyceride level, and insulin resistance. They suggested that fetal malnutrition leads to an impairment of the hypothalamic-pituitary-adrenal axis that may cause altered cortisol secretory patterns throughout life. Also, malnutrition is suggested to lead to β-cell maldevelopment which predisposes to β-cell failure later in life.

A recent study demonstrated that there is an inverse association between fetal glycolated hemoglobin (FGH) of a newborn and its birth weight; that is, low birth weight newborns have a higher percentage of FGH. Fetal glycolated hemoglobin was quantified as a surrogate of fetal glycemia, which possibly reflects insulin resistance [29].

References

1. Eckel RH, Grundy SM, Zimmet P. The metabolic syndrome. Lancet 2005;365:9468–9415.
2. Reaven GM. Banting Lecture: role of insulin resistance in human disease. Diabetic 1988;37:1595–1607.
3. Ford ES, Giles WH, Mokdad AH. Increasing prevalence of the metabolic syndrome among US adults. Diabetic Care 2004;27:2444–2449.
4. Ford ES, Giles WH, Deiltz WH. Prevalence of the metabolic syndrome among US adults: study of NHANES. JAMA 2002;287:356–359.
5. Cameron AJ, Shaw JE, Zimmet PZ. The metabolic syndrome prevalence in worldwide populations. Endocrinol Metab Clin North Am 2004;33:351–375.
6. Ramachandran A, Snehalatha C, Satyavani K, et al. Metabolic syndrome in urban Asian Indian adults—a population study using modified ATPIII criteria. Diabetes Res Clin Pract 2003;60:199–204.
7. Gupta A, Gupta R, Sarna M, et al. Prevalence of diabetes, impaired fasting glucose and insulin resistance syndrome in an urban Indian population. Diabetes Res Clin Pract 2003;61:69–76.
8. Deepa R, Shanthirani CS, Premalatha G, et al. Prevalence of insulin resistance syndrome in a selected south Indian population—the Chennai Urban Populations Study 7 (CUPS-7). Indian J Med Res 2002;115:118–127.
9. Llannie-Parikka P, Eriksson J, Lindstrom J, et al. Prevalence of metabolic syndrome and its components. Diabetic Care 2004;27:2135–2140.
10. Azizi F, Salehl P, Etemadi A, et al. Prevalence of metabolic syndrome in an urban population: Tehran. Diabetes Res Clin Pract 2003;61:29–32.
11. Hu G, Qiau Q, Tuomilehto J, et al. Prevalence of metabolic syndrome and its relation to all-cause and CV mortality in the nondiabetic European men and women. Arch Intern Med 2004;164(10):1066–1076.
12. Dallongerville J, Cottel D, Arveiler D, et al. The association of metabolic disorders with the metabolic syndrome is different in men and women. Ann Nutr Metab 2004;48(1):43–50.
13. Poulsen P, Kyvik KO, Beck-Nielsen H. Genetic vs. environmental etiology of the metabolic syndrome among male and female twins. Diabetologia 2001;44(5):537–543.
14. Pangiotakos DB, Pitsauus C, Chrysohoou C, et al. Impact of life-style habits on the prevalence of the metabolic syndrome among Greek adults from the ATTICA Study. Am Heart J 2004;147(11):106–112.

15. St. Onge MP, Jassen I, Heymsfield SB. Metabolic syndrome in normal weight Americans: new definition of the metabolically obese normal-weight individual. Diabetes Care 2004;(9):222–228.
16. Cooks S, Weitzman M, Auinger P, et al. Prevalence of metabolic syndrome from adolescents for the 111 NHANE Survey 1988–1994. Arch Pediatr Adolesc. 2003;157:821–827.
17. Malhotra S, McElroy S. Association between metabolic syndrome and psychiatric disorder. Pri Psychiatr 2003;10;37–44.
18. Meigs JB, Wilson PW, Nathan DM, et al. Prevalence and characteristics of the metabolic syndrome in the San Antonio Heart and Framingham Offspring Studies. Diabetes 2003;52:2160–2167.
19. Dandona P, Aljada A, Chaudhuri A, et al. Metabolic syndrome. A comprehensive perspective based on interactions between obesity, diabetes, and inflammation. Circulation 2005;111:1448–1454.
20. Aljada A, Ghanim H, et al. Evidence for a potent antiinflammatory effect of rosiglitazone. J Clin Endocinol Metab 2004;89:2728–2735.
21. Pessin JE, Saltiel AR. Signaling pathways in insulin action: molecular targets of insulin resistance. J Clin Invest 2000;106:165–169.
22. Krentz A, Baily CJ. Type 2 Diabetes in Practice, 2nd ed. London: Royal Society of Medicine Press, 2005:P13–29.
23. Czech MP, Corvera S. Signaling mechanisms that regulate glucose transport. J Biol Chem 1999;274:1865–1868.
24. Hales CN, Ozanne SE. For debate: fetal and early postnatal growth restriction leads to diabetes, the metabolic syndrome and renal failure. Diabetologia 2003;4:1013–1019.
25. Yarbrough DE, Barrett-Connor E, Eritz-Silverstein D, et al. Birth weight, adult weight, and girth as predictors of the metabolic syndrome in post menopausal women: the Rancho Bernardo Study. Diabetes Care 1998;21(10):1652–1658.
26. Neel JV. Diabetes mellitus: a "thrifty" genotype rendered detrimental by "progress." Am J Hum Genet 1962;14:353–362.
27. Bavdekar A, Yajnik CS, Fall CH. Insulin resistance syndrome in 8 year-old Indian children: small at birth, big at 8 years, or both. Diabetes 1999;48:2422–2429.
28. Phillip DIW, Barker DJ, Fall CH, et al. Elevated plasma cortisol concentration: a link between low birth weight and in the insulin resistance syndrome. J Clin Endocrinol Metab 1998;83:757–760.
29. Pftab T, Slowinski T, Godes M, et al. Low birth weight, a risk for CVD in later life is associated with elevated fetal glycosylated Hb (FGH) at birth. Circulation 2006;114:1687–1692.
30. Balkan B, Charles MA, Drivsholm et al. Frequency of the WHO metabolic syndrome in European cohorts, and an alternative definition of an insulin syndrome. Diabet Metab 2002;28:364–376.
31. Aguilar-Salinas CA, Rojas R, Gomez-Pevez FJ, et al. Analysis of the agreement between the WHO criteria and the NCEP-III definition of metabolic syndrome. Diab Care 2003;26:1635.
32. Hales CN, Barker DJ. Type 2 diabetes mellitus: the thrifty phenotype hypothesis. Diabetologia 1992;35:595–601.

Chapter 2
Components of Metabolic Syndrome

Q: What are the components of the metabolic syndrome?
The metabolic syndrome is a constellation of interrelated risk factors of metabolic origin—metabolic risk factors that appear to directly promote the development of cardiovascular disease (CVD) or atherosclerotic CVD (ASCVD). Reaven [1] defined the metabolic syndrome as a clustering of cardiovascular (CV) risk factors and metabolic abnormalities. There are two major interacting causes of metabolic origin: obesity and endogenous metabolic susceptibility. The latter is typically manifested by insulin resistance.

The National Cholesterol Education Program's (NCEP) Adult Treatment Panel (ATP-III) reported six components of the metabolic syndrome that relate to CVD [2]:

- Abdominal obesity
- Insulin resistance with or without glucose intolerance
- Atherogenic dyslipidemia
- Raised blood pressure
- Proinflammatory state
- Prothrombotic state

These components of the metabolic syndrome form a group of underlying, major, and emerging risk factors (Table 2.1). According to ATP-III, underlying risk factors for CVD are obesity (particularly central obesity), physical inactivity, and atherogenic diet; the major risk factors are cigarette smoking, hypertension, elevated low-density lipoprotein (LDL) cholesterol, low high-density lipoprotein (HDL) cholesterol, a family history of premature coronary heart disease (CHD), and aging; and emerging risk factors are elevated triglycerides, small LDL particles, insulin resistance, glucose intolerance, proinflammatory state, and prothrombotic state. The underlying risk factors, give rise to the metabolic risk factors. Metabolic factors consist of those factors that apparently have direct effect on

TABLE 2.1. Components of metabolic syndrome

1. Insulin resistance/hyperinsulinemia
2. Obesity, particularly visceral type
3. Glucose intolerance/type 2 diabetes
4. Hypertension
5. Dyslipidemia: elevated triglycerides, reduced HDL cholesterol, increased small, dense LDL cholesterol, increased remnant lipoproteins, increased apoB-III, reduced apoA-III
6. Prothrombotic state: increased PAI-1, increased fibrinogen, increased von Willebrand factor
7. Inflammatory state (i.e., CRP, TNF-α, IL-6)
8. Vascular abnormalities i.e., microalbuminuria, endothelial dysfunction
9. Leptin and adiponectin
10. Hyperuricemia

CRP, C-reactive protein; HDL, high-density lipoprotein; IL, interleukin; LDL, low-density lipoprotein; PAI-1, plasminogen activator inhibitor-1; TNF-α, tumor necrosis factor-α.

atherosclerotic disease, which are atherogenic dyslipidemia, hypertension, elevated plasma glucose, a prothrombotic- and proinflammatory states. Other factors that increase the likelihood of the metabolic syndrome include cardiovascular disease, hypertension, polycystic ovary syndrome, nonalcoholic fatty liver disease, acanthosis nigricans, non-Caucasian ethnicity, sedentary lifestyle, age >40 years, a history of gestational diabetes or glucose intolerance, or a family history of type 2 diabetes, hypertension, or cardiovascular disease. When diabetes becomes overt, the CVD risk increases steeply. Metabolic syndrome is associated with an increased risk of a variety of disease outcome, which include diabetes, peripheral arterial disease, CVD, fatty liver and nonalcoholic steatohepatitis, polycystic ovary syndrome, cholesterol gallstones, asthma, sleep disorders (sleep apnea), and some forms of cancer. The risk of CHD and diabetes with metabolic syndrome are greater than those for simple obesity. The factors most implicated in metabolic syndrome are nonesterified fatty acids (NEFAs), inflammatory cytokines, plasminogen activator inhibitor-1 (PAI-1), adiponectin, leptin, and resistance.

Components of the metabolic syndrome included in various diagnostic criteria are insulin resistance/hyperinsulinemia, glucose disturbance (glucose intolerance, impaired fasting glucose

(IFG), impaired glucose tolerance (IGT), type 2 diabetes), obesity, dyslipidemia, high blood pressure, and microalbuminuria. Insulin resistance is accompanied by many other alterations that are not included in the diagnostic criteria for the metabolic syndrome [3]. These include an increase in apolipoprotein B (ApoB), and C III, uric acid, prothrombic factors (fibrinogen, PAI-1), serum viscosity, asymmetric dimethylarginine, homocysteine, white blood cell count, or proinflammatory cytokines, or the presence of microalbuminuria (not in all criteria), nonalcoholic fatty liver disease/or nonalcoholic steatohepatitis, obstructive sleep apnea, or polycystic ovary disease—all are associated with insulin resistance. Other components that have some role to play include genetic inheritance, sedentary lifestyle, advanced age, hyperleptinemia, increased oxidative stress, and sleep apnea.

INSULIN RESISTANCE

Insulin resistance can be defined as the state in which a normal amount of insulin produces a subnormal biological response. The term *insulin resistance* usually refers to the resistance to the metabolic effects of insulin, including the suppressive effect of insulin on endogenous glucose production, the stimulatory effects of insulin on peripheral (predominantly skeletal muscle) glucose uptake and glycogen synthesis, and the inhibitory effects of insulin on adipose tissue lipolysis. Even before fasting hyperinsulinemia develops, postprandial hyperinsulinemia exists. Fasting hyperinsulinemia in the presence of a normal or elevated plasma glucose level implies insulin resistance. In up to 25% of healthy individuals, unrecognized insulin resistance of a severity similar to that in subjects with glucose intolerance or type 2 diabetes has been seen. While its significance is uncertain, the prevalence of CV risk factors is known to increase with increasing plasma insulin concentration. There are a variety of factors that contribute to insulin resistance, including the distribution of body fat (and total fat mass), the role of free fatty acids (FFAs), adipocytokines, proinflammatory mediators, and genetic factors. Insulin resistance may be secondary to obesity but can have genetic component as well.

Today the potential ramifications of impaired insulin action are recognized by clinicians ranging from endocrinologists to cardiologists. Central to this expanding interest is Reaven's hypothesis that tissue resistance to the effects of insulin is a factor linking non–insulin-dependent diabetes mellitus (NIDDM), essential hypertension, and CHD. Reaven has argued that tissue insulin resistance is the primary initiating defect that leads to compensatory hyperinsulinemia and atherogenic risk factors. Reaven [1], in his 1988 Banting lecture at the American Diabetic Association, focused on the importance of insulin resistance and a related cluster of metabolic abnormalities that were associated with an increase in CAD (coronary artery disease). This cluster included resistance to insulin-stimulated glucose uptake, glucose intolerance, hyperinsulinemia, increased very low density lipoprotein (VLDL) triglyceride, decreased HDL cholesterol, small, dense LDL particles, and hypertension. He suggested the possibility that resistance to insulin-stimulated glucose uptake and hyperinsulinemia were involved in the etiology of the metabolic abnormalities and the clinical classes associated with them. Reaven suggested that the clustering might explain the high prevalence of CVD in individuals with type 2 diabetes.

Insulin resistance usually precedes the onset of type 2 diabetes and contributes to the development of hyperglycemia. The degree to which glucose tolerance deteriorates in insulin-resistant individuals varies as a function of both the magnitude of the loss of in vivo insulin action and the capacity of the pancreas to compensate for this defect. There is a compensatory increase in insulin secretion in an effort to maintain normal blood glucose. As the compensatory mechanism fails to overcome tissue insulin resistance, hyperglycemia ensues. Therefore, individuals with insulin resistance have hyperinsulinemia together with normoglycemia or hyperglycemia. It is therefore clear that resistance to insulin-mediated glucose uptake is a common phenomenon present in the majority of individuals who are glucose intolerant, as well as in a considerable number of people who are apparently healthy. The presence of insulin resistance and hyperinsulinemia per se are independently associated with hypertriglyceridemia. It emphasizes that it is not only insulin resistance that is deleterious but also the compensatory hyperinsulinemia.

Insulin resistance is present in the majority of patients with metabolic syndrome. Insulin resistance and hyperinsulinemia directly cause other metabolic risk factors. The European Group for the Study of Insulin Resistance (EGIR) and the Danish twin register have confirmed that insulin resistance is significantly correlated with the various components of this syndrome. There are various factors that contribute to insulin resistance, including the distribution of body fat, the role of FFAs, adipocytes, proinflammatory mediators, and genetic factors. There could be different types of insulin resistance that may occur in an individual, such as insulin resistance for glucose uptake in skeletal muscle, insulin resistance for glucose release in the liver, insulin resistance for lipolysis in adipose tissue, insulin resistance for amino acid metabolism in skeletal muscle, or any combination of these. People who are overweight, who have a parent or sibling with type 2 diabetes, women who developed gestational diabetes, and some ethnic groups (e.g., South Asians) are at increased risk of insulin resistance.

A number of different altered metabolic states, such as persistent elevation of circulatory glucose, insulin, fatty acids, and cytokines, can lead to peripheral insulin resistance. Most common, however, is a defect at multiple levels. For example, in type 2 diabetes, there are decreases in receptor concentration, in receptor kinase activity, in the concentration and phosphorylation of insulin receptor substrate 1 and 2 (IRS-1 and –2), and in glucose transporter to translocation, and there are defects in intracellular enzymes.

Changes Associated with Insulin Resistance

There are probably several mechanisms of insulin resistance. Some may be due to genetic defects while others are due to acquired factors. However, more than three quarters of cases can be explained on the basis of obesity. Of the several possible mechanisms, one group may be implicated due to insulin antagonists of some kind. Many substances ranging from neurotransmitters (e.g., catecholamine) to hormones (e.g., cortisol, growth hormone [GH]) to cytokines (e.g., tumor necrosis factor-α [TNF-α]) can oppose many insulin actions. When insulin antagonists are the cause, multiple intracellular insulin responsive enzymes can be affected.

Another mechanism of insulin resistance has a common theme of cellular satiety where the cells are overloaded with excess fuel (e.g., carbohydrate derived from overeating) or lipids (as occurs in many cells of obese person), leading to insulin resistance (see Chapter 3). Within cells, there appear to be critical metabolic processes (e.g., accumulation of uridine diphosphate [UDP], glucosamine) that, when saturated, cause multiple changes in cellular enzyme activities that switch off insulin response [4]. There are thus various heterogeneous causes of insulin resistance, and not all people with insulin resistance are the same. Obesity and physical fitness have major roles to play. Inhibition of lipolysis appears to be most sensitive to insulin, while the insulin effect on glucose oxidation is among the least sensitive. Insulin resistance per se is asymptomatic. However, severe insulin resistance may be accompanied by physical signs such as (1) acanthosis nigricans, which involves the axillae and occurs around the nape of the neck; (2) acrochordons—multiple skin tags; (3) hyperandrogenism (e.g., acne, hirsutism, history of menstrual [oligomenorrhea] and conception problems) in women of reproductive age; (4) syndrome-specific features mentioned elsewhere; and (5) acromegaloid features, which may exist in the absence of elevated growth hormone concentration.

OBESITY

Q: What are the classifications of obesity, and how does upper body obesity differ from lower body obesity in its metabolic effects?
More than 65% of adults in the United States are overweight or obese, and one billion individuals worldwide are considered to be overweight. The current concept of adipose tissue is that it is a bona fide organ system with distinct tissue types mediating specific functions such as conserving energy reserves, hormone secretion, and immune regulation [5]. In obesity, there is increased body fat mass, and primarily an increase in the size of fat cells, although the number of fat cells may also be increased, especially in individuals with childhood-onset obesity. The adipocyte is one of the most highly insulin-responsive cell types. Insulin promotes adipocyte triglyceride storing by a number of mechanisms, including promoting differentiation of the preadipocyte to the adipocyte, and, in mature adipocytes, stimulating glucose transport and triglyceride synthesis (lipogenesis) as well as inhibiting lipolysis. Adipocytes are endocrinal glands that secrete important hormones, cytokines, vasoactive substances, and other peptides. Insulin resistance in obesity and type 2 diabetes is manifested by decreased insulin-stimulated glucose transport and metabolism in adipocytes and skeletal muscle and by impaired suppression of hepatic glucose output. These functional defects may result partly from impaired insulin signaling in all three target tissues and in adipocytes, and also from downregulation of the major insulin-responsive glucose transporter GLUT-4.

In obesity, an increased quantity of fat is present in adipose depots and around organs such as the heart and kidneys. Excess lipid is also deposited between cells in nonadipose tissues such as skeletal muscle. Additionally, the deposition of intracellular lipid within adipose cells such as skeletal muscle, heart, and liver is a characteristic feature of the metabolic syndrome, and it has major effects on the metabolic function of the tissue. The classification of obesity is listed in Table 2.2.

Obesity can be classified into upper body type or lower body type. The concept that there are two compartments is now well accepted. These two fat compartments are metabolically quite different. Upper body type (android or male type/central/visceral) is due to excess deposition of fat either intraperitoneally (visceral fat)

TABLE 2.2. Classification of obesity

BMI/waist circumference	Non-Asian	Asians
BMI		
Underweight	<18.5 kg/m^2	<18.5 kg/m^2
Normal	18.5–24.9 kg/m^2	18.5–22.9 kg/m^2
Overweight	25–29.9 kg/m^2	23.0–24.9 kg/m^2
Obese	30.0–39.9 kg/m^2	25.0–34.9 kg/m^2
Morbid	>40.0 kg/m^2	>35.0 kg/m^2
*Waist circumference**		
Men	>102 cm (40 in)	>92 cm (36 in)
Women	>88 cm (>35 in)	>82 cm (32 in)
Waist/hip ratio		
Normal	<1.0 men <0.9 women	<1.0 men <0.9 women

*Ethnicity-based waist circumference, refer to IDF (International Diabetic Federation) Refer Chapter IV.

or subcutaneously. Upper body fat correlates strongly with insulin resistance, but the correlation with visceral fat is even stronger. Visceral fat is distinct from subcutaneous fat. About 80% of total body fat is located in the subcutaneous adipose tissue and 10% is located in visceral adipose tissue. The remainder is located in various other sites such as perirenal and peritoneal areas. Interestingly, visceral fat in men constitutes approximately 20% of total body fat mass as compared to 6% in women. However, this effect is superseded by the fact that 80% of hepatic blood supply is derived from the portal vein, thus enabling greater FFA flux to the liver in the visceral type of obesity than in the subcutaneous type. Also, the total splanchnic blood supply increases postprandially. Thus, the contribution of visceral fat to hepatic FFA uptake and systemic FFA appearance could be significantly more marked in the postprandial than in the fasting state [6].

Lower body obesity (gynoid or female type/peripheral/limb) is characterized by excess deposition fat in the lower part of the abdominal wall and the gluteofemoral area. This type of fat distribution can be readily identified both in women and men. The difference between the two types of obesity can be measured by computed tomography (CT) and magnetic resonance imaging (MRI).

It has been shown that adipose tissue is metabolically active. A study measured glucose uptake using [^{18}F]-fluorodeoxyglucose–positron emission tomography (PET) under conditions of normoglycemia and hyperinsulinemia. The glucose uptake was localized using MRI in abdominal and femoral subcutaneous and visceral adipose tissue before and after treatment. Although the rate of glucose uptake was higher in skeletal muscle fat, there was substantial glucose uptake response to in vivo insulin in subcutaneous fat in the abdominal and femoral regions, and even in visceral and peripheral adipose tissue in the abdominal regions. Also, insulin-mediated glucose uptake was markedly reduced in obese, insulin-resistant individuals [7]. Also, visceral fat cells are more sensitive than subcutaneous cells to the lipolytic effects of catecholamines and less sensitive to the antilipolytic and fatty acid reesterification effects of insulin. This could lead to increased FFA flux in individuals prone to store fat in visceral area.

Nondiabetic women show a very high correlation between central adiposity and insulin resistance ($r = 0.89$). Higher quantities of central obesity are associated with increasing fasting plasma NEFA levels, and lipid oxide and hepatic glucose production. Changes in insulin resistance in people gaining or losing weight are significantly correlated with changes in visceral but not subcutaneous adipose tissue depots [8]. Total body adipose tissue and subcutaneous adipose tissue are significantly correlated with each other, and it is not always possible in obese people to determine which adipose tissue is the independent correlate to a metabolic event.

The waist/hip ratio has been used to estimate the ratio of visceral adipose tissue to subcutaneous adipose tissue. Correlating the anthropomorphic data with either a CT scan or MRI indicates that waist circumference alone is a better surrogate for central obesity than the waist/hip ratio. The waist circumference reflects both abdominal subcutaneous adipose tissue and abdominal visceral adipose tissue and is a general index of central (truncal) fat mass. It has been shown that women too with upper body obesity are more insulin resistant, hyperinsulinemic, glucose resistant, and dyslipidemic than those with lower body obesity. Visceral obesity is most common in South Asians and Mexican Americans as compared with whites of European origin, Chinese, and blacks. Whether these differences are caused by diet, lack of physical activity, genetic factors, or a combination of these is yet to be proven.

Visceral obesity is strongly associated with metabolic abnormalities, such as dyslipidemia, hyperinsulinemia, insulin resistance, and glucose intolerance. The limbic-hypothalamic-pituitary-adrenal axis in patients with visceral obesity is hypersensitive. It has been suggested that visceral obesity can be the result of abnormal cortisol regulation with an augmented stress response. The increased quantity of cortisol secretion plays a role in central obesity and insulin resistance. It has been proposed that central obesity may be due to overexpression of 11β-hydroxysteroid dehydrogenase type 1 (11β-HSD-1) in adipose tissue, leading to increased activity of 11β-HSD-1 [9]. If so, peroxisome proliferation–activated receptor-γ (PPAR-γ) ligand, which significantly reduces 11β-HSD-1 activity in vitro and in vivo and preferentially reduces abdominal adipose tissue, should be the drug of choice for South Asians. Asian Indians have an unexpectedly high percentage of body fat relative to body mass index; there is a proportionate increase in visceral fat. They are markedly insulin resistance and hyperinsulinemic. Among Asian Indians visceral, not subcutaneous, adipose tissue volume is associated with insulin resistance, hyperinsulinemia, and dyslipidemia, and may account for the increased prevalence of CVD and diabetes [10]. In contrast, leptin levels correlated with subcutaneous and total (not visceral) adipose tissue [10].

Visceral adipose tissue has been proposed as the major determinant of insulin resistance/metabolic syndrome and CV complications of obesity, while the subcutaneous fat compartment is the most critical determinant of insulin sensitivity. Increased visceral fat is associated with and may account for the changes in peripheral and hepatic insulin sensitivity seen in obesity. Also, there is differential gene expression between visceral and subcutaneous fat deposits. Visceral obesity is associated with increases in both liver and intramuscular fat. Visceral adipose tissue is measured as a percentage of total body fat. Intraabdominal fat (IAF) is relatively insensitive to insulin and has high lipolytic activity. An important feature of upper body obesity is an unusually high release of NEFA from adipose tissue because it is more metabolically active than subcutaneous fat, with a high rate of triglyceride turnover. This contributes to accumulation of lipid in sites other than adipose tissue such as in muscle and liver (fatty liver or nonalcoholic steatohepatosis). It deteriorates insulin resistance, alters liver metabolism, and predisposes to insulin resistance, dyslipidemia, and finally type 2 diabetes. Fatty liver is even more strongly linked to insulin resistance and to the abnormalities of VLDL metabolism than is whole body adiposity. The features of obesity/overweight and insulin resistance provide a significant risk for developing type 2 diabetes.

c-Jun Amino Terminal Kinase

Recent study suggests that adipose tissue may play a role in inflammation as shown by c-Jun amino terminal kinase (JNK-1) mice studies. JNK-1 can interfere with insulin action and it can also be activated by proinflammatory cytokines such as TNF-α, as well as FFAs [11]. Studies examining JNK-1 and -2 knockout mice have supported the data providing evidence that obesity is associated with abnormally elevated JNK activity, mainly provided by the JNK-1 present in adipose tissue, liver, and muscle. Tumor necrosis factor-α and FFAs associated with insulin resistance activate JNK, which in turn phosphorylates IRS-1 at serines. Impaired regulation of insulin receptor and reduced tyrosine phosphorylation of the IRS proteins may contribute significantly to peripheral insulin resistance and β-cell failure [11]. Our present knowledge indicates that JNK-1 is an important component of the biochemical pathway responsible for obesity-induced insulin resistance in vivo, and further human genetic mutation of JNK activity is associated with the development of type 2 diabetes [12]. However, analysis of JNK-1 represents a potential therapeutic target for treatment of obesity, insulin resistance, and type 2 diabetes.

DYSLIPIDEMIA

Q: How do atherogenic dyslipidemic changes occur in the metabolic syndrome?
The dyslipidemia in metabolic syndrome may be caused by (1) overproduction of VLDL ApoB-100, (2) decreased catabolism of ApoB containing particles, or (3) increased catabolism of HDL-ApoA-1 particles. The major cause of raised plasma triacylglycerol level in nondiabetic individuals is an increase in the hepatic VLDL-triacylglycerol secretion rate secondary to insulin resistance and the resultant hyperinsulinemia. The primary defect most likely is the inability to incorporate FFAs to triglycerides by the adipose tissue (i.e., inadequate esterification), resulting in reduced fatty-acid trapping and consequent reduced retention of fatty acids by adipose tissue. Moreover, similar reduced retention of FFAs is also caused by insulin resistance.

The increased flux of FFAs from peripheral tissues (i.e., adipose tissue) to the liver in insulin resistance condition stimulates hepatic triglyceride synthesis and secretion of triglyceride-rich VLDL, as well as ApoB production in the liver. Insulin suppresses production of large VLDL particles. $VLDL_1$ does not have any effect on the production of the smaller $VLDL_2$ fraction. A decrease in the HDL cholesterol level is due to increased catabolism, related to insulin resistant state. Increased catabolism is related to the pool of triglyceride-rich lipoprotein (mainly VLDL). The increase of plasma triglyceride-rich lipoproteins drives, through cholesteryl transfer protein (CETP), the transfer of triglycerides from triglyceride-rich lipoproteins to HDL, resulting in the formation of triglyceride-rich HDL particles. A low HDL cholesterol level is due to changes in HDL composition and the metabolism of HDL cholesterol particles rich in triglycerides becomes a suitable substrate for hepatic lipase whose activity is enhanced in the insulin-resistant state and type 2 diabetes, leading to increased catabolism of HDL particle. The loss of triglyceride results in a small HDL particle that is filtered by the kidney, resulting in a decrease in ApoA and HDL levels. Additionally, glycation of HDL cholesterol particles occurs in type 2 diabetes and may reduce binding to its receptor. Besides an increase in the loss of apoA, there is evidence that insulin may promote ApoA gene transcription. Hence insulin resistance may be associated with reduced ApoA biosynthesis.

There may be other contributing factors to low HDL cholesterol. One possibility is that even persons with normal fasting triglyceride level have impaired postprandial responses to dietary fat, and that increased cholesteryl ester transfer protein-mediated lipid exchange occurs during the postprandial state. Altered lipid flux in the liver attributable to insulin resistance may reduce hepatic production of ApoA. Another possibility is that insulin resistance may cause destabilization of adenosine triphosphate (ATP) binding cassette A1 transporter protein, a key molecule that mediates the transfer of cellular phospholipids and cholesterol to ApoA for the formation of mature and functional HDL particles. It is noted that mutations in the ATP binding cassette A1 transporter are associated with Tangier disease, which is characterized by low HDL cholesterol [13]. When there is insufficient cholesterol efflux, ApoA is rapidly cleared from the circulation by the kidneys, resulting in a low HDL cholesterol level in plasma. HDL cholesterol has antioxidant, antiinflammatory effects.

Similar to the changes in HDL composition, LDL cholesterol composition and metabolism is also modified. If fasting triglycerides are >2.0 mmol/L (177 mg/dL), invariably all individuals have the dominant presence of small, dense LDL [3]. This alteration of LDL composition is due to relative depletion of cholesterol (unesterified and esterified) and phospholipids with either no change or an increase in LDL triglyceride. This alteration in composition is an independent risk factor for CVD. However, this change often coexists with other concomitant changes of lipoprotein and the presence of other risk factor. The preponderance of small, dense LDL instead of large buoyant LDL also confers increased risk. This does not mean that large buoyant LDL is not atherogenic, but rather that the small, dense LDL molecule is more so. Increased FFA flux to the liver causes enhanced production of ApoB-containing rich VLDL [3]. Normally insulin inhibits secretion of VLDL into the circulation. However, when insulin resistance occurs, increased flux of FFAs to the liver enhances hepatic triglycerides synthesis. This result is partly due to the effect of insulin on the degradation of ApoB. Yet, insulin is also lipogenic, increasing the transcription and enzyme activity of many genes that relate to triglycerides biosynthesis. Also, insulin resistance can diminish the level of lipoprotein lipase in the peripheral tissues (i.e., in adipose tissue more than in muscle), resulting in overproduction of VLDL more than triglycerides.

The ApoB protein, present as one molecule per lipoprotein particle, appears to be more important. First, lipoprotein particles without ApoB are not atherogenic. Second, ApoB has multiple proteoglycan binding domains, which increase the retention of the particle in the subendothelial matrix [4]. Finally, physicochemical and composition characteristics, such as resistance factors against oxidative stress, are likely to be important in reducing the modification of lipoprotein particles. Oxidative modification of ApoB containing lipoproteins converts them to a suitable substrate for macrophage uptake and foam cell formation in the process of atherosclerosis [4].

Remnant Lipoproteins

Q: What is the significance of postprandial lipidemia?
In the presence of insulin resistance, the antilipolytic effect of insulin is weak [13]. This could be the reason that raised FFAs are seen postprandially. It is possible that individuals with metabolic syndrome with normal fasting triglyceride frequently have an abnormal postprandial response to dietary fat. There is a continuous increase of plasma FFAs, which results in an 8-hour plasma FFA concentration that remains above fasting level. Moreover, insulin resistance has two important effects on chylomicron remnant metabolism, the principal lipoprotein formed postprandially. First, it downregulates LDL receptor expression, and second, it increases hepatic cholesterol synthesis and VDRL secretion [13]. These effects enhance competition between chylomicron and VDRL remnants for hepatic receptors, hence impairing the uptake of chylomicron remnants by this pathway. Another reason may be that the disturbance of triglyceride postprandially may relate to the cholesterol homoeostasis [13]. The hepatic cholesterol synthesis and intestinal cholesterol absorption are responsible for the cholesterol content in the liver. The increased intestinal

cholesterol absorption reduces hepatic cholesterol synthesis and as a result the secretion of VLDL decreases and the LDL receptor is upregulated. The upregulation of LDL receptor may increase the removal of both chylomicron and VLDL remnants. In the postprandial state, in the metabolic syndrome, the increased hepatic cholesterol synthesis and decreased intestinal cholesterol absorption do not result in a decrease in the catabolism of triglyceride remnants [13]. Abnormal postprandial lipidemia is related to CVD.

Remnant lipoproteins are found elevated in the metabolic syndrome. They are formed in the postprandial state and may add to CV risk. Remnant proteins and small, dense LDL may increase in response to a low-fat diet, but whether the overall effect is detrimental or not is not clear. In fact, remnant lipoproteins are more than balanced by a low-fat diet because of the reduction in total plasma cholesterol and body weight. Postprandial levels of lipids are important, as humans spend considerable time in the postprandial state due to their eating habits. It is therefore crucial to assess the impact of postprandial levels of lipids on health and disease. It is in the postprandial state when atherogenic lipoproteins are formed, such as chylomicron and the VLDL remnant (which may add to CV risk). Also, frequent eating during the day creates a continuous postprandial state, which predisposes to the modification of other stable lipoproteins such as LDL.

The HDL cholesterol level is also reduced in the presence of triglyceride-rich lipoproteins. If the lipolytic removal of postprandial lipoprotein is slow, fewer building blocks for de novo synthesis of HDL components are formed. Therefore, the atherogenic lipoprotein phenotype (ALP) is formed after long-standing moderate hypertriglycidemia or repeated episodes of augmented postprandial hypertriglycidemia, which affects lipoprotein adversely in terms of both quality and quantity. There is some evidence that markers of exaggerated postprandial lipidemia are associated with the severity of CVD. The postprandial triglycidemic effect of a low-fat diet can be countered by moderate physical exercise or by inclusion of long-chain n-3 polysaturates in the diet. Fish oils reduce fasting and postprandial triglycerides as well as remnant lipoproteins. This may have beneficial cardiovascular effect.

Q: How does particle size of lipids exert its atherogenicity?

Individuals with metabolic syndrome typically do not have elevated levels of LDL cholesterol or it may be mildly elevated. Interestingly, the atherogenic potential of LDL cholesterol is defined not only by the cholesterol level of this class of lipoprotein but also by the size and numbers of LDL particles. Recent nuclear magnetic resonance

(NMR) has been used to directly measure the size and concentration of plasma lipoproteins. An increase in LDL particles number, especially small LDL, parallels an increase in metabolic syndrome components in both men and women in the Framingham Heart Study population. Although an increased number of small LDL particles as a single measure is highly predictive of the metabolic syndrome, a higher number of small LDL particles was not associated with an increase in CVD event rate. There is increasing evidence that the size of the LDL particle plays a crucial role in its atherogenic properties. Particle size is determined by flotation rates after ultracentrifugation procedures. The higher the fasting triacylglycerol level, the greater will be the postprandial accumulation of triacylglycerol-rich lipoproteins (i.e., VLDL, chylomicron remnants, and VLDL remnants) in the nondiabetic individual.

The LDL particle could be larger (diameter >25.5 nm; pattern A) or smaller LDL (diameter ≤25.5 nm; pattern B). Individuals with pattern B LDL have higher plasma triacylglycerols and a lower HDL level than those with pattern A LDL. Individuals with small, dense LDL particles (pattern B) are comparatively insulin resistant, glucose intolerant, hyperinsulinemic, hypertensive, and hypertriglyceridemic, and have low HDL cholesterol. There is evidence that individuals with elevated small, dense LDL particles have a higher incidence of CHD and more accelerated progression of coronary lesions [4]. The exact mechanism is not understood. However, it is proposed that smaller particles (1) penetrate the endothelium more easily, (2) are more likely to be deposited in the arterial wall than larger particles, (3) bind more avidly to proteoglycans [4], (4) are more toxic to the endothelium, (5) adhere well to glycosaminoglycans, (6) are more likely to oxidize, and (7) are more selectively bound to scavenger receptors on monocyte-derived macrophages.

Also, small, dense LDL particles most commonly occur with elevated triglycerides, low HDL, and insulin resistance—components of the metabolic syndrome. Research suggests that it is possible to change the LDL particle size from small to large by reducing triglycerides and normalizing insulin sensitivity. In clinical practice, lipid-lowering drugs such as bile-binding resins, niacin, and fibrates are reported to alter particle favorably.

Small, Dense Low-Density Lipoproteins
There is a significant reduction of LDL catabolism associated with reduced LDL production (secondary to decreased LDL catabolism). Therefore, there is reduced turnover of their LDL particles, with a reduction of catabolism leading to increased LDL cholesterol

plasma residence time, which is likely to enhance cholesterol deposition in the arterial wall [4]. The formation of small, dense triglyceride-rich LDL particles (known as subclass B) is complex and is thought to be due to a genetic trait, but the major gene responsible is not fully known. Plasma triglycerides, which are affected by dietary intake, play a crucial role. The presence of small, dense LDL particles mainly appears to be related to hyper-triglyceridemia. Small, dense LDL particles are produced by sequential interaction between LDL particles and triglyceride-rich lipoprotein, during which cholesteryl esters contained in the core of the LDL particle are exchanged for triglycerides by CETP [4]. The CETP transfers cholesterol from LDL to VLDL while simulta-neously exchanging triglyceride in the opposite direction. Triglycerides entering the LDL particle are hydrolyzed by hepatic lipase. The gradual exchanges deplete LDL of cholesterol, resulting in a reduction of the size of the particle. The protein content of the particle remains constant but becomes denser. This process is slow when there are few triglycerides. Hence, the formation of LDL small, dense particles is dependent on the level of triglyceride-rich lipoprotein because there is a positive correlation between plasma triglycerides and small, dense LDL. The particles are associated with increased cardiovascular risk. Increased LDL oxidation is another metabolic change that increases atherogenicity. Glycated LDL particles are easily oxidized and are preferentially taken up by macrophages to the formation of foam cells.

Low-fat diets may elevate triglyceride levels and subsequently cause a reduction in the LDL size. However, the benefits of a low-fat diet remain, and the net effect on CV risk remains unclear. The increase of small LDL particles in response to a low-fat diet may be genetically determined [4]. A combination of 4-week inter-vention with a low-energy, low-fat diet, together with physical activity, reduced body weight, plasma triglycerides, and the num-ber of small, dense LDL particles in a group of obese men with type 2 diabetes [14].

High-Density Lipoprotein Subtractions

Individuals with small-dense LDL particles also have small, dense HDL particles, because the lipid components of the two lipopro-tein species have a common metabolic pathway with shared and co-coordinated regulated gene products [4]. In HDL there are two apolipoproteins, ApoA-I and ApoA-II, and several other minor components such as ApoE and ApoC. The two main terminologies by which HDL is often described are based on size or density (i.e., HDL_2 and HDL_3, subdivided into HDL_{2a}, HDL_{2b}, HDL_{3c}) or on apolipoprotein composition (i.e., lipoprotein containing either only ApoA-I [LpA-I] or both ApoA-I and ApoA-II [LpA-I:LpA-II). The presence of larger HDL is dependent on a low concentration of triglycerides. Both HDL cholesterol and HDL$_2$ cholesterol are strongly inversely related to plasma triglyceride levels. Low-fat diets either reduce or have no effect on the plasma HDL$_2$ level, but physical exercise increases its level.

Remnant-Like Particles

It is known that remnants of triglyceride-rich lipoproteins (TRLs) are atherogenic but there is no consensus of opinion on its definition, nor is there a standardized method for its measurement. Recent studies have used the monoclonal anti-ApoB antibody J1-H for this purpose [4]. The initial observation showed that the properties of the J1-H antibody exclude binding of chylomicrons and chylomicron remnants. Also, ApoB-100 containing TRLs with an excess of ApoE appears to be excluded from binding to the antibody. This is important, as the abundance of ApoE on the surface of a lipoprotein is a characteristics feature of the remnant [4]. The number of remnant-like particles is elevated in various hyperlipidemic states, and the level is normally higher in individuals with CHD than in controls.

PROINFLAMMATORY STATE

Q: How are inflammation, obesity, and insulin resistance interrelated?

Hotamisligil et al first described the association between inflammation and obesity [24] and laid the first foundation for this concept. They supported the close association between obesity and inflammation, as they showed that adipose tissue expresses proinflammatory mediators (e.g., TNF-α, interleukin-6 [IL-6], C-reactive protein [CRP], migration inhibitor factor [MIF]). They also showed that the inflammatory mechanism may have a role to play in insulin resistance and pathologies associated with increased cardiovascular risk [24]. This proved the concept that the inflammatory cytokine TNF-α was a mediator in insulin resistance. Macrophages in the obese tissue may produce proinflammatory factors and they may also regulate the secretory activity of adipocytes. Mononuclear cells in obesity express an increased number of proinflammatory cytokines and related factors, and have been shown to be in an inflammatory state. Also, these cells have a significantly increased binding of nuclear factor κB

(NF-κB), the proinflammatory transcriptor of p65 (Rel A), the major protein component of NF-κB. These cells also express diminished amount of I-κBβ, the inhibitor of NF-κB. All this supports the hypothesis that obesity is an inflammatory state.

Most recent studies have linked insulin resistance with TNF-α, CRP, and IL-6, and each has shown that a measure of inflammation is predictive of type 2 diabetes. Insulin has an antiinflammatory effect on endothelial and mononuclear cells by increasing levels of I-κB. This causes reduced levels of proinflammatory cytokines such as TNF-α, IL-6, and adhesion molecules (i.e., vascular cell adhesion molecule [VCAM] and intercellular adhesion molecule [ICAM]) and chemokines (i.e., CRP). However, this pathway can be blocked by insulin resistance and some cytokines allow atherogenesis to occur.

The proinflammatory state is recognized clinically by elevation of CRP, which is commonly present in individuals with the metabolic syndrome. Multiple mechanisms underline the elevation of CRP. One reason is obesity, because excess adipose tissue releases inflammatory cytokines that may elicit CRP levels. It has been suggested that metabolic syndrome is associated with chronic, low-grade inflammation, and it possibly aggravates the symptoms. Inflammatory cytokines induce insulin resistance of both adipose tissue and muscle. Increased production of inflammatory cytokines strengthens the connection between obesity and inflammation. Individuals with insulin resistance show evidence of low-grade inflammation even without the increase of total body fat. The presence of an inflammatory state indicates a higher risk of an acute cardiovascular syndrome. Most of the components of the metabolic syndrome are positively associated with inflammatory markers and are independent of age, gender, physical activity, smoking, and body mass index (BMI). Proinflammatory stimuli like lipopolysaccharide (LPS) and proinflammatory cytokines (i.e., TNF-α and IL-6), cause phosphorylation of I-κB) and subsequent translocation of NF-κB to the nucleus. Intranuclear NF-κB induces the transcription of proinflammatory genes like TNF-α, IL-6 and IL-1β, ICAM-1, and VCAM-1, and cytokines like monocyte chemoattractant (chemotactic) protein-1 (MCP-1) and CRP.

No drug is presently available for reducing raised CRP associated with inflammatory state. However, several drugs used to treat other metabolic risk factors have been found to reduce CRP (e.g., statins, nicotinic acid, fibrates, angiotensin-converting enzyme inhibitors [ACE-Is], thiazolidinedione (TZDs). At present these drugs are not recommended specifically to reduce proinflammatory state.

Q: What is the value of C-reactive protein in metabolic syndrome and CVD?

C-reactive protein is an acute-phase reactant inflammatory marker produced and released by the liver under the stimulation of cytokines including IL-6, IL-1, and TNF-α. It is a reliable measure of underlying systemic inflammation and a strong predictor of future myocardial infarction and stroke. In most people CRP concentrations were found to be <1.0 mg/dL. Han et al [16] reported that CRP was a significant predictor of metabolic syndrome only in women but not in men in the Mexico City Diabetes Study. High-sensitivity C-reactive protein (hs-CRP), a marker of inflammation, is an independent predictor of future risk of CV events among healthy individuals, as well as among patients with acute coronary syndrome. Besides, hs-CRP adds prognostic information on all future CV risk at all levels of LDL cholesterol, at all Framingham risk scores. C-reactive protein is strongly associated with the metabolic syndrome and with CVD. Low-grade inflammation is indicated by an increased level of inflammatory mediators. It is now widely accepted that small increases in CRP, within the high normal range, predict the likelihood of developing CV events independent of the severity of atherosclerosis. The studies of different ethnic groups have shown that CRP is independently associated with the metabolic syndrome [17]. In this study, CRP was independently related to insulin sensitivity in healthy subjects, and increased concomitantly with an increase in the number of components of the metabolic syndrome. A prospective, epidemiological evaluation of CRP in the Women's Health Study found that elevation of CRP predicted the risk of future diabetes even after multivariate adjustment for the common measures of adiposity (BMI and waist circumference).

Recent evidence suggests that hs-CRP plays a major role in the physiological process associated with the metabolic syndrome [18]; hs-CRP levels of <1 mg/L, 1 to 3 mg/L, and >3 mg/L should be interpreted as low, moderate and high risk, respectively, even when applied to those already defined as having the metabolic syndrome. The prospective data suggest that measurement of CRP adds clinically to the prognostic information regarding the metabolic syndrome [18].

C-reactive protein elicits direct proatherogenic and proinflammatory effects and has been shown to act as a direct mediator of endothelial dysfunction. C-reactive protein at a level that is accepted as predicting CV events directly reduces endothelial cell nitric oxide (NO) production by destabilizing endothelial NO synthase (eNOS) transcription. By reducing NO release, CRP inhibits angiogenesis and stimulates endothelial cell apoptosis. C-reactive protein also promotes the release of the potent endothelium-derived contracting factor endothelin-1 (ET-1), which is partly responsible for CRP-induced upregulation of adhesion molecule ICAM-1. C-reactive protein also upregulates MCP-1 release. The evidence shows that CRP also enhances NF-κB upregulation in atherosclerosis. In the atherogenic process, CRP directly enhances native LDL uptake into macrophages, a process that is ET dependent. Angiotensin-II is a known proinflammatory molecule that can enhance atherosclerotic process at the level of endothelium and vascular smooth muscle (VSM).

Ridker et al [18] showed that a CRP level of >3 mg/L had almost identical prognostic value in terms of CVD event-free survival over 8 years, as did a full assessment of metabolic syndrome. C-reactive protein was also observed to add prognostic information to the metabolic syndrome definition. In the Jupiter trial, women who had CRP levels of <3 mg/L without the metabolic syndrome had the best vascular survival, whereas those with ≥3 mg/L with the metabolic syndrome had the worse vascular survival [19]. In the Framingham Offspring Study, CRP and the metabolic syndrome were independent predictors of new CVD events [20]. There is some recent evidence that CRP concentration varies among ethnic groups, naturally leading to the idea that CRP level could be used to assess CVD risk in different ethnic groups [21]. Asian Indians have a higher CRP as compared to white Europeans, and this ethnic difference disappeared when adjusted for either BMI or waist circumference. Hispanic women have a higher CRP than European white women in the National Health and Nutrition Examination Survey (NHANES) 1999-2000 study. The NHANES-III study found the highest CRP among black men and Mexican-American women and in all ethnic groups (European whites, blacks, and Mexican Americans), but Mexican Americans had the highest CRP of these ethnic groups [22].

The components of the metabolic syndrome—abdominal obesity, high blood pressure and high fasting glucose—are modestly associated with elevated levels of CRP. The CRP level also correlates with other components of the metabolic syndrome that are not easily measured in clinical practice, including fasting insulin, microalbuminuria, and impaired fibrinolysis. A recent study assessed the interrelationship among CRP, the metabolic syndrome, and incident CV events among 14,719 healthy women, and found that 24% had the metabolic syndrome; these subjects were followed for 8 years to assess the incidence of myocardial infarction (MI), stroke, coronary revascularization, and CV death. It was noted that at all levels of the metabolic syndrome, the level of CRP improved the risk prediction for future CV events [18]. Additionally, the CRP level was highly predictive even among those with the full metabolic syndrome at study entry. C-reactive protein is stimulated by IL-6 and is positively correlated with insulin resistance, obesity, and endothelial dysfunction [23].

Q: What are the proinflammatory adipokinases produced by adipose tissue and what is their implications in insulin resistance?

Two forms of adipose tissues have been found: brown (BAT) and white (WAT). In humans, significant amounts of BAT are found only in neonates, and there is conversion between the two types. It is the WAT type that is important in the expression of various inflammatory factors. Adipocyte size is highly correlated with indicators of systemic insulin resistance, dyslipidemia, and risk for development of type 2 diabetes. Monocyte-derived macrophages that reside in adipose tissue might partly be responsible for the expression of proinflammatory cytokines locally and in systemic circulation (Table 2.3).

TABLE 2.3. Adipose tissue–derived factors

Adipokines	Functions
TNF-α	Interferes with insulin signaling (induced insulin resistance), activates inflammatory pathways, including NF-κB
Leptin	Affects satiety and appetite signals to brain to regulate body fat mass
Interleukin-6	Stimulates liver production of CRP, promotes inflammation
PAI-1	Functions as potent inhibitor of fibrinolytic pathway
Adiponectin	Affects regulation of insulin sensitivity and role in inflammation
Adipsin	Functions in the activation of complement system
Angiotensinogen	A precursor of a vasoconstrictor, proinflammatory, and pro-oxidant mediator
ASP	Acts as adipocyte autocrine factor
Resistin	Negative affect on glucose transfer
PPAR γ	Regulates body cell gene expression in human subcutaneous adipose sites

ASP, acylation stimulating protein; CRP, C-reactive protein; PAI-1, plasminogen activator inhibitor-1; PPAR γ, peroxisome proliferators-activated receptor gamma; TNF-α, tumor necrosis factor-α.

Tumor Necrosis Factor-α

Tumor necrosis factor-α is expressed as a 26-kDa transmembrane cell-surface protein and cleaved into the circulatory biologically active 17-kDa form. It has multifunctions and is involved in the development of insulin resistance. It is produced by a variety of cells such as monocytes/macrophages (residing in adipose tissue). Tissue macrophages are derived from monocytes in the blood. Hotamisligil et al [24] showed that neutralization of TNF-α with soluble TNF-α receptors result in restoration of insulin sensitivity. Tumor necrosis factor-α is hyperexpressed in obesity (correlated with fat depot mass) and is a mediator of insulin resistance. It is implicated in the causation of insulin resistance by a variety of mechanisms.

Tumor necrosis factor-α increases hormone-sensitive lipase (HSL) activity, resulting in increased lipolysis and FFA release from adipose tissue to the liver. hormone-sensitive lipase interferes with insulin signaling and IRS protein formation at the postreceptor level. This impairs insulin-mediated glucose uptake by adipocytes through downregulation of insulin-responsive glucose transport (GLUT-4). Tumor necrosis factor-α reduces body weight by decreasing appetite, increasing lipolysis, and promoting adipocyte apoptosis [25]. It also downgrades PPAR expression. It also plays a crucial role in suppressing the expression of most adipocyte-specific genes (i.e., *PPAR*). Experimental studies have shown a positive correlation between TNF-α and obesity [26]. There is also an association between TNF-α expression in adipose tissue and features of insulin resistance in obese and diabetic models. Tumor necrosis factor-α induced serine phosphorylation of IRS-1, which in turn causes the serine phosphorylation of the insulin receptor [3]. This prevents the normal tyrosine phosphorylation of the insulin receptor and thus interfered with insulin signal transduction. Interleukin-6 and TNF-α have been shown to induce suppressor of cytokines signaling-3 (SOC-3), which interferes with tyrosine phosphorylation of the insulin receptors and IRS-1 and causes proteosomal degradation of IRS-1 [3]. This reduces the activation of Akt (protein kinase B), which causes the translocation of the insulin-responsive glucose transporter, GLUT-4, to plasma membrane. It also induces phosphorylation of the enzyme NOS and its activation to generate NO. Tumor necrosis factor-α appears to have a catabolic role in adipose tissue. It stimulates lipolysis, decreases lipoprotein lipase (LPL) activity, and reduces activity of lipogenic enzyme LPL via suppression at the messenger RNA (mRNA) and protein level. Other adipokines are discussed in the answers to the following questions.

Leptin

Q: What is the mode of action of leptin and its clinical implications?
Leptin is a protein that is predominantly secreted by adipose
tissue. It plays a role in fat metabolism and closely correlates
with insulin resistance and other markers of the metabolism,
independent of total adiposity. The defective leptin action may
contribute to insulin resistance in the metabolic syndrome. It
circulates in the blood as proteins of 146 amino acids with a
molecule mass of 16 kDa. Leptin is a hormone that responds to
metabolic effects on peripheral tissues as a satiety signal. It
controls appetite and regulate body weight via receptors in the
brain. The receptors of leptin have been found in the hypothalamus and surrounding brain regions, which supports the
idea that leptin has a centrally mediated effect on appetite,
metabolism, and other endocrine systems involved in the star-
vation process [27]. Additionally, leptin receptors have also
been found in other tissues such as adipose tissue, skeletal
muscle, the liver, the pancreas, and tubular renal cells. This
may explain leptin's other roles, such as that it regulates glucose uptake into skeletal muscle tissue and adipose tissue as
well as being implicated in the development of insulin resistance. A decrease in body fat leads to a decrease in hormone
level, which in turn stimulates food intake by increasing the
appetite. In increased body fat, increased levels of leptin reduce
the appetite by acting on the brain. By this process it regulates
body weight. The plasma levels of leptin are significantly correlated with adipose tissue mass. Its level is increased in obesity
and decreased after weight loss. Leptin is proinflammatory and
platelet proaggregatory. Hyperleptinemia may contribute to the
proinflammatory state in obesity and to atherogenesis in the
long term.

Leptin is the product of the obese *(ob)* gene originally identified as defective and responsible for the obesity syndrome in
ob/ob mice [28]. The leptin receptor (LE PR) belongs to the class 1
cytokine receptor family, which includes the receptor for IL-6
leukemia inhibitory factor (LIF), granulocyte colony-stimulating
factor (G-CSF), and glycoprotein 130 (gp 130). The leptin signal
is transmitted mainly through the Janus kinase (JAK) signal
transducers and activators of transcription (STAT) signal transduction pathway, and terminated by induction of suppressor of
cytokine signaling (SOCS-3). Also, the leptin signal can modulate
the expression or activity of a number of insulin targets, including IRS-1, mitogen-activated protein (MAP) kinase, extracellular

regulated kinase (ERK), p38 MAP kinase, Akt (protein kinase B, PKB), P kinase, and phosphatidylinositol (PI)-3-kinase [29]. The concept of leptin resistance is based on the fact that raising the leptin levels beyond the threshold of transport does not intensify the signal of satiety to the hypothalamus. The threshold to leptin may be further lowered by defects in the pathway of leptin signal transduction. Therefore, several defects in insulin signaling are associated with severe constant hunger, leading to obesity. It is postulated that leptin resistance can develop in the face of high circulating levels of hormone. Indeed, resistance to the central anorectic effect of leptin develops rapidly in the face of nutrient excess. Resistance to leptin and insulin are closely linked in humans.

The mechanism of action of leptin in skeletal muscle may be via regulation of adenosine monophosphate (AMP)-activated protein kinase, which has been shown to increase fatty acid oxidation, reduce ectopic fat deposits in nonadipose tissue, and improve insulin sensitivity [30]. Deregulation of this system (AMP kinase [AMPK] signaling) has been suggested as a common feature that may cross-link some metabolic derangements seen in the metabolic syndrome. Although the exact mechanism is not known, it is likely that the effect of leptin may be via the central nervous system (CNS)-mediated increase in sympathetic nervous system activity, as well as for a direct effect on the target tissues [30]. It is also proposed that, leptin being a cytokine, it can together with CRP, IL-6, and IL-1 induce an acute-phase reactant to regulate inflammatory processes through direct activation of leptin signaling in the target cells [31].

It is likely that leptin stimulates the production of MCP-1 and reactive oxygen species (ROS). Leptin induces mitochondrial superoxide production and MCP-1 expression in aortic endothelial cells by increasing fatty acid oxidation via protein kinase, which in turn increases monocyte infiltration and foam cell accumulation in the injured artery, and induces the synthesis of ET-1, promoting vasoconstriction. Leptin signaling activation in platelets further increases platelet aggregation around the atherosclerotic lesion.

The identification and sequencing of the mouse obese *(ob)* gene by Friedman's group [32] in 1994, and the isolation of its product, leptin, have provided new insights into the relation between obesity and insulin resistance. In homozygous *ob/ob* mice, the mutation of the ob gene results in increased food intake, reduced energy expenditure, elevated insulin and cortisol levels, and subsequently in massive obesity and NIDDM [32]. The *ob* gene encodes a protein, leptin, which is produced only in fat cells and secreted into the blood. Administration of leptin corrects the multiple metabolic disturbances. In humans, insulin resistance is associated with raised plasma leptin concentrations independent of body fat mass. A causal relationship between leptin and insulin sensitivity has been suggested, and this may help explain the pathogenesis of the insulin resistance syndrome [33].

Insulin resistance also occurs in apparently lean subjects. It is proposed that lean insulin resistance individuals have a greater amount of body fat than do lean insulin-sensitive subjects. Alternatively, their body fat distribution may be different. Insulin sensitivity has also been proposed to be another determinant of leptin concentrations, possibly through stimulation of leptin secretion from adipose cells by insulin. However, the association between insulin and leptin is difficult to assess because adipose tissue affect both leptin levels and insulin sensitivity. Elevated leptin levels have been proposed as an independent risk factor for CHD in a large prospective study, the West of Scotland Coronary Prevention Study (WOSCOPS) [34].

Leptin has been shown to be antilipogenic in some tissues, and it upregulates fatty acid oxidation [6]. Leptin deficiency states such as lipodystrophic syndromes are associated with huge nonadipose tissue fat accumulation due to increased lipogenesis and reduced fatty oxidation. Hyperleptinemia is associated with obesity, insulin-resistant states, and type 2 diabetes, suggesting that leptin resistance, not leptin deficiency, may be the responsible pathophysiology. Fasting serum level of leptin are correlated with the subcutaneous, not the visceral, adipose volume [35].

Obese individuals seem to be resistant to a high leptin level, so the leptin does not signal effectively to the brain to reduce appetite. Leptin resistance possibly plays a role in extra-adipose tissue fat deposition and lipotoxicity. It could also result in increased fatty acid availability to tissues. Elevated levels of plasma FFA cause relative suppression of leptin release by adipose tissue, which impairs leptin signaling in insulin-resistant states [6]. It is possible to regain leptin sensitivity with weight loss or nutrient restriction, which may have a favorable implication for insulin action.

Adiponectin

Q: What is the clinical importance of adiponectin in the metabolic syndrome?
Adiponectin is a 30-kDa adipose-specific protein that appears to increase insulin sensitivity. It is secreted in adipose tissue, also

known as the adipocyte complement-related protein of 30 kDa (Acrop30), AdipoQ, and gelatin-binding protein of 28 kDa (GBP28), apM1. It is the product of the human *apM1* gene and is a 247 amino acid protein consisting of an N-terminal collagenous region and a C-terminal globular domain [27]. It enhances insulin sensitivity and inhibits many steps in the inflammatory process. In the liver it diminishes both the hepatic gluconeogenesis enzyme and the rate of endogenous glucose synthesis. In the muscle, adiponectin increases glucose transport and increases fatty acid oxidation, an effect partly due to AMPK. Adiponectin is antiinflammatory, and its level falls in the presence of weight gain and obesity [36]. Adiponectin plasma concentrations are reduced in patients with type 2 diabetes and cardiovascular disease, and correlate inversely with both insulin resistance and obesity. Adiponectin stimulates fatty acid oxidation, decreases plasma triglycerides, and improves glucose metabolism by increasing insulin sensitivity.

Adiponectin reduced the triglyceride content of muscle and liver in obese mice by increasing the expression of fatty acid oxidation and energy dissipation in muscle [6]. A recent prospective study and meta-analysis suggests that any association between adiponectin level and CHD risk is unlikely to be strong [37]. Adiponectin despite being driven solely from adipose tissue is paradoxically reduced in obesity. Circulating adiponectin levels range from 0.5 to 30 mg/mL and reportedly are almost 1000-fold higher than circulating levels of other hormones such as insulin and leptin.

The mechanism leading to decreased adiponectin level in obesity is not fully understood. Adiponectin is inhibited by insulin and TNF-α. Hence, hyperinsulinemia caused by obesity-induced insulin resistance, together with enhanced TNF-α expression, may contribute to reduced adiponectin secretion. It is also suggested that visceral fat may produce some unidentified substances that destabilizes adiponectin mRNA [38]. Adiponectin not only has a direct beneficial effect on insulin sensitivity, fat, and glucose metabolism, but also may provide benefit within the vasculature, mediated through its ability to increase the phosphorylation and activation of AMP/malonyl–coenzyme A (CoA) signaling and to decrease the inflammatory pathway via reduction of NF-κB activity [39].

The NF-κB/Rel family of proteins are inducible transcription factors that play a major role in regulating the expression of a wide variety of genes associated with cell proliferation, inflammation, and cell survival [40]. Therefore, the net effect of increased adiponectin signaling is enhanced fatty oxidation, and increased glucose utilization, reduced endogenous glucose production, and decreased inflammation [40].

Acrop30 has been shown to have an inhibitory effect on the NF-κB signaling pathway, and as NF-κB is involved in the transcription of many proinflammatory cytokines, this may be a possible mechanism through which acrop30 reduces insulin resistance. However, the acrop30 receptor has not yet been identified, and the signaling pathway through which acrop30 produces its effects still remains unclear. Genetic polymorphism of the adiponectin gene is associated with increased incidence of insulin resistance and diabetes. There does not seem to be any acute effect of macronutrient excess or deprivation on the adiponectin levels, and chronic energy restriction (which promotes insulin action) increases the adiponectin levels. Also, a raised baseline level of adiponectin is associated with a significant reduction of diabetes type 2.

The plasma level of adiponectin in Caucasians and Pima Indians are negatively correlated with percentage of body fat and plasma insulin levels, and are positively correlated with insulin-mediated glucose uptake [37]. Adiponectin has been shown to reverse insulin resistance associated with both lipoatrophy and obesity [40]. Increased expression of the adiponectin gene also has been shown to increase insulin sensitivity, improve glucose tolerance, and decrease NEFA concentration [41]. A depot-specific pattern of mRNA expression of adiponectin in adipose tissue has been observed, implicating an inverse correlation with adiponectin expression and visceral adiposity [5].

Adiponectin has been suggested to act in the brain to increase energy disposal and decrease body weight [5]. This effect is particularly synergistic with that of leptin. It is proposed that adiponectin circulates in two forms: a relatively low-molecular-weight (LMW) hexamer and a high-molecular-weight (HMW) multimeric structure. The ratio of these two oligometric forms has been shown to correlate more tightly with insulin action than does total circulatory adiponectin level [41]. The HMW structure has been suggested to be the active form of adiponectin, and that it acts favorably on glucose metabolism at liver levels.

Reduced level of adiponectin in CHD is indicative of its antiatherogenic effect. Also, adiponectin increases endothelial production of nitric oxide and inhibits growth-factor–induced vascular smooth muscle cell proliferations. It inhibits TNF-α–induced expression of VCAM-1, E-selectin, and ICAM-1, and suppresses the effect of TNF-α to induce the adhesion of monocyte THP-1 cells to cultured endothelial cells. Adiponectin also suppresses TNF-α–induced inflammatory changes in the endothelial cells by blocking inhibitory NF-κB phosphorylation and NF-κB activation. Therefore, adiponectin has a potent antiinflammatory and atheroprotective effect in vascular tissue in addition to its insulin-sensitizing effects in tissues involved in glucose and lipid metabolism. A reduced level of adiponectin in visceral adiposity also contributes to endothelial vascular dysfunction in addition to its role in inducing insulin resistance and glycemic disturbance, leading to typical features of the metabolic syndrome [42]. It has been suggested that low adiponectin may be a marker for athero-sclerosis and CHD [36]. Indeed, in contrast to associations with CHD previously observed in the same participants in the British Heart Foundation Research Group for a range of established risk factors (e.g., smoking, blood pressure, blood lipids) and emerging markers (e.g., CRP), the inverse associations observed with adiponectin levels were comparatively modest and not statistically significant [36]. However, adiponectin levels are more strongly related to type 2 diabetes than CHD.

Adiponectin is reduced in Asian-Indian men and healthy African-American boys. It is also proposed that ethnic differences in the concentration of both leptin and adiponectin might con-tribute to the differential ethnic risk for the metabolism syndrome as well as CVD. Adiponectin is also linked to the development of dyslipidemia, as is PC-1, which is a membrane glycoprotein that reduces insulin-stimulated tyrosine kinase activity and thus exerts its role in insulin resistance.

Resistin

Resistin is a 10-kDa adipose tissue-specific hormone. Resistin (F1ZZ3) belongs to a family of cysteine-rich C-terminal proteins known as resistin-like molecules (RELM; RELM α F1ZZ1 and RELM β F1ZZ2) of F1ZZ, which are suggested to be involved in inflammatory process [43]. Resistin has been suggested as the potential link among obesity, insulin resistance, and type 2 diabetes by some [43], while others have not found any such reliable link. Although *in vivo* resistin appears to affect insulin action, there is increasing uncertainty about its significance.

Acylation Stimulating Protein

Acylation-stimulating protein (ASP) is a small, basic serum protein capable of stimulating triglyceride synthesis in fibroblasts and adipocytes. It is identical to C3adesArg, the inactive fragment of the complement anaphylatoxin peptide, C3a, and it is generated by mature adipocytes secreting the three complement proteins: com-plement protein C3, factor B, and factor D (adipsin) [4]. Acylation-stimulating protein may act as an adipocyte autocrine factor and play a crucial role in the metabolism of adipocytes [4]. Studies show that there is a quantitative correlation of ASP or ASP precursors with adipose tissue mass and concentration of circulatory hormones, carbohydrates, and lipids. The level of ASP or ASP precursors is increased in obese and diabetic individuals but is decreased in subjects with lipodystrophy and anorexia nervosa [44]. The level also correlates with plasma insulin, glycosylated hemoglobin, triglycerides, and fatty acids. The association of ASP with hypertension and CVD has also been shown [44]. Furthermore, the ASP levels are higher in obese women than in obese men, which may be due to higher ASP production from subcutaneous adipose tissue (which is more prominent in women). It has been suggested that dysregulation of the ASP pathway may increase postprandial lipemia and alter lipoprotein profiles, hence predisposing to the metabolic syndrome and increased CV risk. The plasma level of ASP is higher in the obese than in lean individuals. How ASP deficiency or resistance induces metabolic and vascular disorders is not clear.

Acylation-stimulating protein also may play a role in (1) C3adesArg, promoting synthesis of triglycerides by stimulating fatty acid incorporation in adipocytes; (2) promoting translocation of GLUT-1, -3, and -4, and stimulating adipocyte glucose uptake; (3) activating diacylglycerol acyltransferase, which participates in triglyceride synthesis; (4) increasing lipogenesis; and (5) inhibiting activity of HSL and HSL-mediated lipolysis by stimulating FFA reesterification

Macrophage and Monocyte Chemoattractant Protein-1
Macrophage, and monocyte chemoattractant (chemotactic) protein-1 (MCP-1) are chemokines that recruit monocytes to the sites of inflammation and in adipose tissue. They are mainly expressed and released from the nonadipose tissue. It has been shown that their expression is increased in rodent obesity [45]. The increased level of MCP-1 is associated with increased infiltration of macrophages in the adipose tissue and enhanced release of proinflammatory cytokines (e.g., IL-1, IL-6). Adipose tissue–expressed MCP-1 may have endocrinal or autoparacrinal action. In adipose tissue it may induce insulin resistance via impairing insulin-stimulated insulin receptor tyrosine phosphorylation and insulin-stimulated glucose uptake by the adipose cells and inhibit adipogenesis [45]. Recently, the chemokine MCP-1 was also shown to impair adipocyte sensitivity [46].

Coagulation and Complement Factors
Fibrinogen and PAI-1 are increased in obesity. Plasminogen activator inhibitor-1 (PAI-1) is mainly produced by the liver, but an

appreciable quantity is also synthesized by adipose tissue. There is a close association among plasma PAI-1 levels, visceral adiposity, and CV risk, indicating that PAI-1 may play a role in thromboembolic complications in obesity. There seems to be an independent role of adipose tissue–derived factors in immune regulation. The link between adipose tissue and the complement system drew attention initially due to the presence of C3 deficiency in subjects with partial lipodystrophy. Differentiated 3T3–F442A adipocytes synthesize and secrete complement D (adipsin) [46]. In humans, unlike rodents, blood levels of adipsin are increased in obese subjects and decreased with fasting or in conditions of lipoatrophy [47]. A role for the complement system in adipocyte biology was also indicated when ASP was identified as stimulating triglyceride synthesis in fibroblasts [46].

Steroids and Glucocorticoids

Adipose tissue does not synthesize steroid hormones *de novo*, but is involved in steroid interconversion. The ratio of active to inactive glucocorticoids (cortisol vs. cortisone) in fat depots is regulated by 11β-HSD-1 [46]. 11β-HSD-1 is regulated by insulin, and this affects the local metabolism of glucocorticoids in adipose tissue. There is a close association between chronic hypercortisolism in Cushing syndrome, and central obesity, insulin resistance, diabetes, hypertension, and CV mortality. The experimental studies in mice show the role of adipose-tissue–derived glucocorticoids in metabolism and CV regulation [48]. Mice with transgenic overexpression of 11β-HSD-1 in adipocytes have normal circulating levels of corticosterone, but the local glucocorticoid level is increased in adipose tissue [49]. These mice develop visceral obesity and features of the metabolic syndrome such as insulin resistance, impaired glucose tolerance, dyslipidemia, hypertension, and hepatic steatosis [48,49].

Q: What is it in the inflammatory state that results in the causation of insulin resistance?

An Inflammatory Hypothesis

There is increasing evidence that the relationship between inflammation and insulin resistance is not merely correlative but actually causative [47]. Inflammation might impair insulin action through various mechanisms. The main messenger in immune responses is cytokines. Of the many cytokines, TNF-α, IL-1, and IL-6, which are produced by monocytes and macrophages, activate a number of cell functions that define their role in immune responses. These cytokines increase vascular permeability and expression of adhesion molecules by endothelial cells in the arterial wall, enabling the infiltration of granulocytes and lymphocytes into the site of injury and infection where they help with the clearance of pathogens. The liver is an important target for the action of cytokines. It responds to their signals by synthesizing acute-phase proteins (e.g., CRP), which are required for repair and recovery. C-reactive protein has several direct effects on the initiation or progression of vascular disease. In particular, it appears to be involved in several stages of plaque development. It may promote the recruitment of monocytes into the intima, mediate LDL uptake by macrophages, and induce the expression of cell adhesion molecules (Fig. 2.1).

Tumor necrosis factor-α correlates with fat depot mass. Therefore, obesity may be an important factor in linking obesity with inflammation. Conversely, insulin resistance may also promote chronic inflammation. Insulin itself has potent acute antiinflammatory effects, including in ROS generation, MCP-1, and PAI-1, and also has some action on hepatic protein synthesis, increasing the synthesis of albumin but suppressing that of acute-phase proteins [50]. The insulin resistance may enhance production of CRP, fibrinogen, and other acute-phase proteins. Also, endothelial cells are insensitive, and insulin resistance correlates with endothelial dysfunction. Hyperinsulinemia can increase the expression of ICAM-1 and thus helps macrophage recruitment into the endothelium [50].

Inflammatory Markers as Predictors of Metabolic Syndrome
Most studies have focused on the value of CRP and other markers in predicting the development of type 2 diabetes. The studies show that CRP, IL-6, and some other inflammatory markers predict the development of diabetes in different ethnic groups. However, the predictive power of CRP is the strongest. Elevated CRP also predicted the progression of IGT to type 2 diabetes and the development of gestational diabetes. In the Kuopio Ischemic Heart Disease Risk Factors (KIHD) study, men with CRP level >3 mg/L had a severalfold higher age-adjusted risk of developing metabolic syndrome (NCEP definition; odds ratio [OR], 3.2; 95% confidence interval [CI], 1.9–5.5; World Health Organization [WHO] definition: OR, 3.4; 95% CI, 2.0–6.1) or diabetes (OR, 4.1; 95% CI, 2.1–8.0) than men whose levels were <1.0 mg/L [51]. However, after adjustment of potentially confounding lifestyle factors and factors related to insulin resistance, CRP was no longer significantly predictive of the metabolic syndrome. Therefore, it is likely that some of the risks are mediated through obesity and insulin

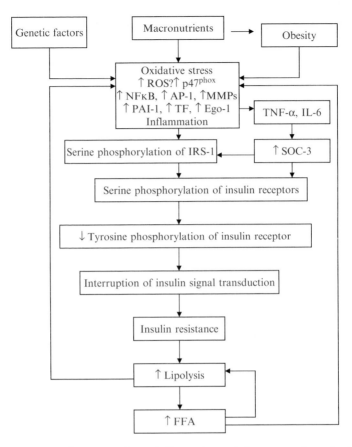

FIGURE 2.1. Pathogenesis of metabolic syndrome: inflammatory hypothesis. IL, interleukin; MMP, matrix metalloproteinase; NF, nuclear factor; PAI-1, plasminogen activator inhibitor-1; ROS, reactive oxygen species; TF, tissue factor; TNF-α, tumor necrosis factor-α. (From Dandona et al. [36].)

resistance. Low adiponectin levels predict an increased incidence of type 2 diabetes and also development of gestational diabetes. It was shown in the Données Epidémiologigues sur le Syndrome d'Insulino-Résistance (DESIR) Cohort Study, that nucleotide polymorphism may independently affect the development of several components of the metabolic syndrome [52].

Insulin Resistance: An Inflammatory Hypothesis
It is postulated that the inflammatory state leads to insulin resistance. Obesity is a very common cause of insulin resistance, and

the underlying mechanism is through ectopic lipid accumulation. However, obesity is also associated with a chronic inflammatory response manifested classically by production of various cytokines and activation of inflammatory signaling pathways. Inflammatory response may induce insulin resistance by two different pathways. First, activation of inflammatory signaling in intermediates may be directly involved in serine phosphorylation of IRS-1 within insulin-sensitive cell types such as hepatocytes and myocytes and thus induce insulin resistance [53]. Second, inflammatory cell infiltration within adipose tissue may be involved in altering adipocyte lipid metabolism (e.g., TNF-α promotes lipolysis) as well as altering cytokine production by adipose tissue, which may in turn have a downstream effect on other metabolically important tissues. Tumor necrosis factor-α is thought to induce insulin resistance by way of involving serine phosphorylation of IRS-1.

Hotamisligil et al showed that TNF-α induced serine phosphorylation of IRS-1, which induced the serine phosphorylation of the insulin receptor. These processes prevented the normal tyrosine phosphorylation of the insulin receptor that interferes with insulin signal transduction [26]. Hotamisligil's group [54] found another inflammatory serine kinase to be involved in inducing serine phosphorylation of IRS-1, called Jun kinase 1 (JNK-1). This showed that c-JNK can interfere with insulin action in cultured cells and are activated by inflammatory cytokines and FFAs that have been implicated in the development of type 2 diabetes. Furthermore, an absence of JNK-1 results in decreased adiposity, significantly impaired insulin sensitivity, and enhanced insulin receptor signaling capacity in two different models of mouse obesity. The activity of JNK-1 is correlated with serine phosphorylation of IRS-1 and insulin resistance. Fatty acid–induced serine phosphorylation of IRS-1 might be mediated by another inflammatory signaling intermediate, namely I-κB kinase-β (I-κBK-β) [55].

Suppression of cytokine signaling 3 (SOCS-3) has recently been shown to interfere with tyrosine phosphorylation of the insulin receptor and IRS-1. Suppression of cytokine signaling 3 is another important contributor to the links among obesity, inflammation, and insulin resistance [56]. This study showed that in both obesity and lipopolysaccharide-induced endotoxemia there is suppression of cytokine signaling (SOCS) proteins SOCS-1 and SOCS-3 in liver, muscle, and to a lesser extent fat. This study further shows that SOCS-1 and SOCS-3 act as negative regulators in insulin signaling and serve as one of the missing links between insulin resistance and cytokine signaling. Tumor necrosis factor-α and IL-6 induced SOCS-3, which inhibits insulin signaling. The SOCS family of proteins is thought to participate in negative feedback loops in cytokine signaling.

SOCS-1 and SOCS-3 have been shown to block insulin signaling by ubiquitin-mediated deregulation of IRS-1 and IRS-2 [36]. This, in turn, reduces the activation of Akt (protein kinase B), which normally causes the translocation of the insulin responsive glucose transporter, GLUT-4, to the plasma membrane [35]. Akt-dependent phosphorylation affects the activation of eNOS in endothelial cells and generation of NO. Protein kinase B/Akt2 is an important protein involved in insulin signal transduction. It mediates the phosphorylation and activation of endothelial NOS and NO secretion, and also prevents the mobilization of Rac-1 to the cell membrane, hence preventing superoxide generation. Superoxide generation is dependent on translocation of essential elements of reduced nicotinamide adenine dinucleotide phosphate (NADPH) oxidase such as $p47^{phos,}$ from the cytosol to the membrane [36]. As a result, in the absence of Akt2, there is an increase in the translocation of Rac-1 to the membrane, greater formation of NADPH oxidase complex, and increased superoxide generation and oxidative stress. Akt2 plays an essential role in insulin signaling. A study showed that mice deficient in Akt2 are impaired in the ability of insulin to lower blood glucose because of the defect in the action of the hormone on the liver and skeletal muscle, establishing Akt2 as an essential gene in the maintenance of glucose homeostasis [57].

Deficiency of, or an excess of, certain adipokines may be involved in the pathogenesis of insulin resistance. Their role is discussed in respective adipokines. The Insulin Resistance Atherosclerosis Study found that insulin resistance is significantly associated with higher hs-CRP levels, higher fibrinogen, and higher PAI-1 levels. These elevated PAI-1 and CRP levels predict the development of type 2 diabetes.

Q: What is the evidence that macronutrients induce inflammation?
The recent global explosion of obesity is due to a larger energy intake and physical inactivity. High-carbohydrate diets can increase insulin secretion, which aggravates insulin resistance, especially in obese individuals. This led to the concept that a diet that contains moderate amount of fat (33% to 38% of energy) but rich in unsaturated fatty acids may be more beneficial in the treatment and prevention of insulin resistance more than a low-fat, high-carbohydrate diet. A study concluded that glucose intake stimulates ROS generation and $p47^{phox}$ of nicotinamide adenine dinucleotide phosphate (NADP) oxidase, increases the oxidative load, and causes a fall in α-tocopherol

TABLE 2.4. Effects of 75g-glucose intake

1. Increases superoxide generation by leukocytes by 140% over the basal level.
2. Increases p47^{phox} expression, a subunit of NADPH oxidase
3. Increases intranuclear NF-κB binding
4. Decreases in inhibitor κB (I-κB) expression
5. Increases I-κKα and I-κ (the kinases that phosphorylates I-κBα and I-κBβ
6. Increases AP-1, which regulates the transcription of matrix metallo proteinase
7. Increase in Egr-1 and matrix metalloproteinase 2 and 9, TF, PAI-1

AP-1, activated protein-1; TF, tissue factor.
Source: Dandona et al. [36].

concentration [58]. The effects of a 75-g glucose challenge are listed in Table 2.4.

Macronutrient intake has been shown to induce oxidative stress and proinflammatory changes in the plasma and peripheral mononuclear cells (MNCs) of a normal person. A diet containing large quantities of fat and less of fruits, fiber, and vegetables is common today. It results in an inability of endogenous insulin (secreted in response to the meal intake) to suppress the inflammation initiated by the meal. Further, an equicalorie intake of fat or cream produces the same amount of oxidative stress. Conversely, reduced calorie intake (1000 kcal for 4 weeks) and 24-hour fasting reduces the oxidative stress and inflammatory markers. Recent work shows that fats, particularly saturated, are inflammatory while fruits and vegetables are not. The work of Dandona et al [36] supports the hypothesis that obesity is proinflammatory, and macronutrient intake may induce oxidative stress and the inflammatory process. It was observed that a 900-kcal American Heart Association Step 2 diet–based meal rich in fruits and fibers does not cause significant oxidative stress or inflammation in contrast to the effects of an isocaloric fast-food restaurant meal [1]. It supports the hypothesis that macronutrients may induce inflammation and oxidative stress. Some macronutrients have now been shown to be safe, are not proinflammatory, and do not cause oxidative stress. The intake of vitamin E before a glucose challenge also suppresses oxidative stress and inflammation. Vitamin E intake in individuals with insulin resistance reduces cytokine production by MNCs [1]. α-Tocopherol therapy (AT) supplementation in type 1 diabetic patients has been shown to ameliorate diabetic microvascular complications. α-Tocopherol therapy, in addition to decreasing LDL oxidative susceptibility and platelet aggregation, seems to have appreciable effects on monocyte and endothelial function. α-Tocopherol therapy supplementation in diabetic patients could also result in a reduction in microvascular disease [59]. It is also noted that alcohol and orange juice given in equicaloric amounts do not cause oxidative stress or inflammation [1].

In a study, fat/cream intake of same caloric value resulted in a similar amount of oxidative stress [60]. High caloric intake food in obesity causes a state of chronic oxidative stress and proinflammatory changes, and an inflammatory mechanism interferes with insulin transduction. These alterations contribute directly or indirectly to insulin resistance, which leads to atherosclerosis and type 2 diabetes, if pancreatic β cells fail to respond to an increasing demand of insulin.

A meal from a fast-food restaurant showed an increase in NF-κB and a decrease in I-κB in mononuclear cells, an increase in I-κKα and I-κKβ, and an increase in superoxide radicals generated by MNCs, evidence of a proinflammatory effect [61]. Elevation of FFAs induces inflammation and impairs vascular reactivity in healthy subjects [1]. This study has shown for the first time that an increase in plasma FFA levels acutely causes an increase in the intranuclear NF-κB binding activity and p63 expression (and decreased I-κBβ) in MNCs, as well as ROS generation by MNCs. Clearly, therefore, an increase in FFA level is associated with the induction of proinflammatory changes and oxidative stress. Because elevated FFAs inhibit glucose uptake by insulin-responsive organs, such as skeletal muscle, it has been suggested that FFAs may be the major mediators of insulin resistance.

A study showed the suppressive effect of dietary restriction and weight loss in the obese on the generation of ROS by leukocytes, lipid peroxidation, and protein carboxylation, and the evidence supported both oxidative stress and inflammatory mediators [62]. Similarly, another study showed an inhibitory effect of a 2-day fast on ROS generation by leukocytes and plasma orth-tyrosine and meta-tyrosine concentrations [63]. The expression of p47[phos] was also reduced. All this evidence supports the idea that macronutrient intake is a major regulator of oxidative stress. The superoxide radical produced during oxidative stress is an activator of NF-κB and activated protein-1 (AP-1), both of which are proinflammatory transcription factors;

NF-κB regulates the transcriptional activity of at least 125 genes, most of which are proinflammatory [1], which supports the idea that obesity is proinflammatory. The circulatory mononuclear cells in the obese have been shown to be in a proinflammatory state [1].

A high-fructose diet and a high-fat diet with specific fatty acid composition have each been shown to affect insulin resistance directly. It has been observed that a high-fructose (found in fruits) or high-sucrose diet can cause features of the insulin resistance syndrome. From animal studies, it has been suggested that a high-fructose or high-sucrose diet can induce the elements of insulin resistance [64]. This study found that (1) MNCs in obesity are in a proinflammatory state with an increase in intranuclear NF-κB binding, a decrease in I-κβ in MNCs, and an increase in the transcription of the proinflammatory genes regulated by NF-κB; (2) the plasma FFAs are a modulator of inflammation; and (3) insulin resistance is a function of inflammatory mediators.

It has been proposed that fructose causes hyperinsulinemia and hypertension, but it has not yet been proven. However, a high-fat diet does cause insulin resistance as compared to a low-fat diet [4]. But it is difficult to implicate fat alone, as total energy intake also has an effect, including the role of obesity. Other possible effects include alteration in the physical properties of cell membranes (e.g., membrane fluidity), alteration in insulin receptor binding or activation, and the local effects of muscle triglyceride accumulation [4]. Of the different types of fats, saturated fatty acids have the most harmful effect on insulin action [65]. Certain monosaturated fatty acids (e.g., palmitoleic acid and n-6 polyunsaturates) also have harmful effects. Trans-fatty acids seem to enhance insulin secretion, at least in the short-term, to a greater extent than do *cis*-fatty acids. However, more evidence is needed to confirm this idea. In contrast, isoenergic substitution of long-chain n-3 polyunsaturates (e.g., fish oils) for saturated fatty acids reduces insulin resistance in some studies [65]. Excess alcohol intake seems to have several metabolic effects, including weight gain and direct damage to the pancreatic β cell. Alcohol can also contribute to hypertriglyceridemia and insulin resistance. Some micronutrients have also been implicated in the causation of insulin resistance. A deficiency of chromium, zinc, vanadium, vitamin D, or carnitine causes insulin resistance, and dietary replacement improves it [4]. Chromium, vitamin D, and carnitine deficiency are not common inducers of insulin resistance.

PROTHROMBOTIC STATE

Q: What is the role of fibrinolytic system in the pathogenesis of metabolic syndrome?

Fibrinolysis

The important step in the initiation of fibrinolysis is the conversion of zymogen plasminogen to the enzyme plasmin by tissue-type plasminogen activator (t-PA) and urinary-type plasminogen activator (u-PA). Tissue-type plasminogen activator, u-PA, factor XIIa, and kallikrein are fibrinolytic factors, and PAI-I and antiplasmin are inhibitors of this system. Tissue-type plasminogen activator is released into the circulation from vascular endothelial cells, which are stimulated by various agents, such as nicotinic acid and catecholamine, as well as by exercise. Plasma t-PA levels exhibit a distinct circadian rhythm, being lowest in the morning.

Plasmin needs to bind to fibrin to be effective, and fibrin acts as both a cofactor and a substrate. When a fibrin clot is forming, t-PA and plasminogen bind sequentially to fibrin, thereby providing a situation in which plasmin regenerates rapidly. Furthermore, the original plasminogen, called glu (glutamine) plasminogen, is converted to a more activatable form, lys (lysing) plasminogen, upon fibrin binding. Additional pathways of plasmin generation involve two plasminogen proactivators, one of which is converted to plasminogen activator by factor XIIa and kallikrein, and the other of which (urokinase type; u-PA) is activated by plasmin, thereby producing a positive feedback mechanism.

Plasmin is able to degrade both fibrinogen and fibrin, but only a limited number of accessible lysing sites are available on fibrinogen. A complex series of fibrin and fibrinogen degradation products are generated by the lytic action on free fibrinogen, fibrin monomer, and polymeric cross-linked fibrin [4]. Endothelial cells exert an anticlotting role by (1) providing an intact barrier; (2) releasing prostacyclin (prostaglandin I_2, PGI_2) and nitric oxide, which inhibit platelet aggregation; (3) secreting tissue factor pathway inhibitor; (4) binding thrombin (via thrombomodulin), which activates protein C; (5) displaying molecules on the surface of their plasma membrane; and (6) secreting plasminogen activator.

Vascular endothelium is a major source of t-PA in plasma. Its release is stimulated by a number of mediators including thrombin. Urinary-type plasminogen activator is activated by plasmin. Plasmin degrades fibrin to fibrin degradation products (FDPs) (Fig. 2.2). Plasminogen activator inhibitor-1 inhibits t-PA, u-PA, and activated protein C, thus promoting thrombin generation,

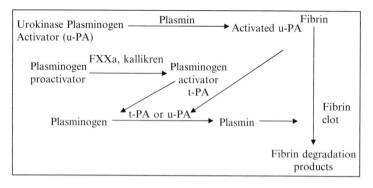

FIGURE 2.2. The fibrinolytic pathway. t-PA, tissue-type plasminogen activator; u-PA, urinary-type plasminogen activator.

platelet aggregation, and fibrin formation. Plasma-derived α_2-antiplasmin also inhibits activated protein C and specifically inactivated plasmin released from clots [4].

Protein C and protein S are major natural anticoagulants in the body and have a powerful role in anticoagulation. The major plasminogen activator is t-PA. Another plasminogen activator is the urokinase type, u-PA, which is synthesized in the kidney and released into the urogenital tract. Intrinsic plasminogen activator such as factor XII and prekallikrein are of minor physiological importance. Inactivators of plasmin such as α_2-antiplasmin and thrombin-activatable fibrinolysis inhibitor (TAFI) also contribute to the regulation of fibrinolysis. α_2-Antiplasmin also inhibits activated protein C and inactivates plasmin released from clots.

Activated protein is generated from its vitamin K–dependent precursor by the action of thrombin; thrombin activation of protein C is augmented when thrombin is bound to thromboplastin, which is an endothelial receptor. Activated protein C destroys factor VI and factor VIII, reducing further thrombin generation.

The fibrinolytic (or thrombolytic) system is the principal effector of clot removal. Tissue factor pathway inhibitor (TFPI), protein C, and antithrombin-III all function to limit clot formation. In this system, plasma proenzyme plasminogen is activated to the active enzyme by protein plasminogen activators. Once formed, plasmin dissolves fibrin. Fibrin is an important initiator of the fibrinolytic process. The presence of fibrin profoundly increases the ability of t-PA to catalyze the generation of plasmin from plasminogen. TAFI is activated by a raised concentration of thrombin formed after clot or thrombin formation. A low concentration of thrombomodulin significantly increases the generation of TAFI by thrombin, whereas high concentrations upregulate fibrinolysis by reducing thrombin generation via activated protein C and hence reducing activation of factor XI thrombin. Activated platelets provide a surface for thrombin's activation of factor XI.

It has been suggested that the clinical markers of prothrombosis should include an increased ratio of fibrinopeptide A (FPA, a small peptide released from fibrinogen) to D-dimer. It has been noted that D-dimer levels are often increased in the presence of active thrombosis [4].

In the fibrinolytic system t-PA antigen and PAI-1 antigen cause impaired fibrolysis, and they are positive risk factors for CHD. Plasma PAI-1 levels are affected by IL-6, and PAI-I is a strong predictor of type 2 diabetes [4]. Interleukin-6 stimulates the production of acute phase-proteins including fibrinogen, CRP, and von Willebrand factor (vWF). Elevated levels of fibrinogen contribute to a prothrombotic state by its marked effect on blood viscosity. Von Willebrand factor is also a CHD risk factor. Its level can be increased by IL-6 stimulation, and its risk is conveyed through its role in coagulation as a cofactor for factor VIII.

Obese patients are prone to coagulation due to increased plasma concentrations of fibrinogen, factor VII, factor VIII, vWF, and several other factors. Also, there is a reduced concentration of antithrombotic factors. Plasminogen activator inhibitor-1 predicts a recurrence of myocardial infarction, and there is an increased PAI-1 concentration in atheromatous plaques. Increased PAI-1 strongly correlates with BMI and fasting insulin levels in type 2 diabetes and also with triglyceride levels in nonobese individuals.

Fibrinogen

An increase in plasma fibrinogen levels is also associated with insulin resistance. Fibrinogen is synthesized in the liver. The data from the insulin resistance atherosclerosis study [66] clearly show that higher plasma fibrinogen levels are independently correlated with fasting plasma insulin and with insulin resistance. Fibrinogen is an acute-phase reactant that is a strong independent predictor of thrombotic CV events. Elevated levels of fibrinogen are also associated with other acute-phase proteins, including CRP, and this could be the expression of an acute-phase response accompanying the inflammatory components of CHD. Therefore, prothrombin and the proinflammatory state appear interrelated. The inflammatory cytokine IL-6 stimulates the production of acute-phase proteins including CRP, fibrinogen, and vWF [4]. A raised level of fibrinogen is a contributing factor for the prothrombotic state through its effect on increased blood viscosity.

Von Willebrand factor, another CHD risk factor, is increased by IL-6 stimulation but then enhances the risk via its role in coagulation, as a cofactor for factor VIII.

Platelets, Insulin Resistance, and Type 2 Diabetes

The platelets contribute to vessel occlusion following the rupture of an atheromatous plaque both indirectly, by promoting vasoconstriction, and directly, through the formation of intravascular thrombosis. The platelets in insulin-resistant individuals are resistance to the action of insulin, NO, and PGI_2, suggesting that platelets aggregation in fact is upregulated in the setting of insulin resistance. It has been suggested that platelet activation is increased in the metabolic syndrome and type 2 diabetes as reflected by increased levels of constituents of platelet granules (β-thromboglobulin and platelet factor) in plasma [4]. The loss of insulin regulation of platelet function in insulin resistance could contribute to the increased atherothrombotic risk associated with metabolic syndrome. In patients with the metabolic syndrome who are at moderately high risk for ASCVD events, aspirin prophylaxis is an alternative option to lower vascular events associated with the prothrombotic state.

Q: What components of the prothrombotic state are relevant in the pathogenesis of the metabolic syndrome and CVD?

A prothrombotic state implies an imbalance between coagulation and fibrinolysis that encourages fibrin deposition and clot formation, such as through an increased sensitivity of platelets to activation or an imbalance in thrombin's different roles. However, a prothrombotic state is not necessarily a prelude to a thrombotic event. A prothrombotic state is characterized by increased PAI-1 and increased fibrinogen, and is associated with metabolic disorders. Although plasma levels of many clotting factors such as VII, VIII, XII, and XIII B-subunit are raised, the fibrinolytic system is relatively inhibited as a result of raised PAI-1.

Hemostatic Mechanism and Insulin Resistance

Insulin resistance is associated with prothrombotic risk factors PAI-1, factors VII, XII, XIII B-subunit, and fibrinogen. Type 2 diabetes is associated with significant suppression of fibrinolysis caused by elevated levels of PAI-1, but the association with insulin resistance is the strongest. The plasma level of PAI-1 in healthy individuals is correlated with the degree of insulin resistance, fasting plasma insulin, and triacylglycerol and HDL cholesterol levels. The *PAI-1* gene possesses a triglyceride-responsive element that may explain this association and enforces a link between diabetes and suppression of fibrinolysis. The familial nature of the link between insulin resistance and thrombosis is supported by similar clustering of risk in the nondiabetic, insulin-resistant, first-degree relatives of patients with type 2 diabetes [67].

Plasminogen activator inhibitor-1 is an inhibitor of fibrinolysis and is found in plasma and in platelets, from which it is released on activation. It inhibits not only t-PA and u-PA, but also protein C, thereby enabling thrombin generation, platelet aggregation, and fibrin formation [4]. Its synthesis is augmented by insulin, proinsulin-like peptide, triglyceride-rich VLDL and lipoprotein particles, endotoxin, IL-6, and oxidized LDL cholesterol. Plasminogen activator inhibitor-1 production is stimulated by insulin [66].

The PAI-1 level is highest in the early morning and reduces gradually in the afternoon. This protein is secreted by adipose tissue, endothelial cells, and hepatocytes. Exposure of hepatocytes to insulin or VLDL enhances PAI-1 release. Proinsulin augments PAI-1 release from both hepatic and endothelial cells. Therefore, there is a strong link among insulin, VLDL, and PAI-1. A reduction in insulin concentration through exercise and weight loss is associated with a fall in PAI-1 activity and VLDL cholesterol [4]. Individuals with the metabolic syndrome have increased levels of PAI-1, vWF, and fibrinogen.

Plasminogen activator inhibitor-1 inhibits the conversion of plasminogen to plasmin, thereby decreasing fibrinolysis. An elevated level shifts the balance of the thrombotic-fibrinolytic system in favor of thrombosis in blood vessels. Metformin or thiazolidinedione (TZD), which decreases insulin resistance, also reduces PAI-1 levels. Plasminogen activator inhibitor-1 is now accepted as a risk factor for CAD. Von Willebrand factor is synthesized and secreted primarily by endothelial cells. Its level correlates with both plasma insulin levels and insulin resistance. The increase in the level of vWF in insulin-resistant states is indicative of endothelial dysfunction and could be associated with an increase in the production of adhesion molecules.

ENDOTHELIAL DYSFUNCTION

Q: What is the pathophysiology of endothelial dysfunction, and how does it relate to insulin resistance and the metabolic syndrome?
Endothelium forms the partition between the arterial wall and the constituents of blood. It plays a crucial role in the regulation of vascular tone, and inhibiting leukocyte adhesions and

platelet aggregation, via its release of mediators such as NO and prostacyclin. Nitric oxide is derived from L-arginine through the action of eNOS. The vasodilatory effect of NO leads to increased circulation to the target organ. Insulin resistance may directly lead to endothelial dysfunction [50]. It has been proposed that insulin resistance predicts atherosclerosis as it alters the permeability barrier function, enhances adhesion molecule expression, increases leukocyte adhesion, impairs endothelium-dependent vasodilator responses, enhances thrombosis, and impairs fibrinolysis. Furthermore, it has been shown that hyperinsulinemia can increase the expression of ICAM-1, increasing macrophage attachment to the endothelium.

Constituents of modified lipoprotein particles, among them certain oxidized phospholipids and short-chain aldehydes arising from lipoprotein oxidation, can induce transcriptional activation of the *VCAM-1* gene mediated in part by NF-κB and proinflammatory cytokines such as IL-1β and TNF-α, which are increased in the metabolic syndrome and induce VCAM-1 expression by this pathway. Thus proinflammatory cytokines may link altered endothelial function to the dyslipidemia of the metabolic syndrome [50].

Endothelial dysfunction associated with oxidative stress predicts CVD. Insulin resistance reduces the production of NO by endothelial cells. The mechanism involves inhibition of PI-3-kinase activation (insulin hypothesis). Insulin normally binds to its receptors and phosphorylates IRS-1, which in turn activates the PI-3-kinase, which plays an important role in both insulin-mediated glucose disposal in adipose tissue and also in NO production by the endothelial cells. The insulin stimulation of PI-3-kinase is reduced in obese individuals and almost absent in type 2 diabetes [27]. This selective insulin resistance leads to enhancement of the mitogenic pathway with increased vascular smooth muscle cell (VSMC) growth and migration and increase in PAI-1 and endothelium [27]. This pathway is present in the vasculature, heart, and kidneys [1]. Elevated plasma NEFAs reduce endothelial-dependent NO production and vasodilatation. It is possible that elevated NEFA, observed in central obesity and insulin resistance, contributes to endothelial dysfunction in the insulin resistance state by impairing NO production and increasing mitotic activity at the endothelial level, and that VSMCs switch the balance toward an atherogenic state. Tumor necrosis factor-α suppresses the expression of NOS. These factors result in abnormalities in endothelial-mediated vasodilatation and vascular reactivity. The abnormalities in vascular reactivity in the obese insulin resistant population can be reproduced by a 900-kcal fast-food restaurant meal [1] (Fig. 2.3).

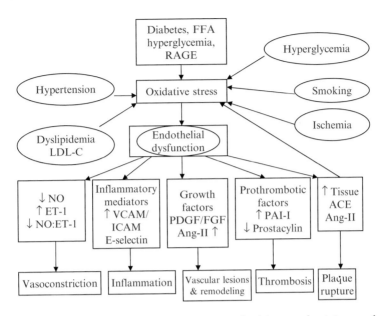

FIGURE 2.3. Important cellular processes involved in vascular injury and atherosclerosis. Ang-II, angiotensin-II; ET-1, endothelin-1; FFA, free fatty acids; FGF, fibroblast growth factor; ICAM, intracellular cell adhesion molecule; NO, nitric oxide; PAI-1, plasminogen activator inhibitor-1; PDGF, platelet-derived growth factor; RAGEs, receptor for advanced glycation end products (promotes inflammation and oxidation, particularly in cells involved in atherogenesis); VCAM-1, vascular cell adhesion molecule-1. (From Staels B. PPARgamma and atherosclerosis. Curr Med Res Opin 2005;21(suppl 1):S13–20.)

Insulin resistance and systolic blood pressure are the principal determinants of endothelial dysfunction in the metabolic syndrome. Hypertension may induce endothelial dysfunction by several pathways, such as through mechanical damage, increased endothelial cell free radical formation, reduced NO bioavailability, or via its proinflammatory effect on VSMCs. Insulin resistance is associated with a weakened endothelium-dependent response that is not augmented by euglycemic hyperinsulinemia [27]. In part the endothelial dysfunction may be due to elevated free fatty acids.

Hyperglycemia promotes endothelial dysfunction and resistance to insulin (glucose hypothesis). An elevated blood glucose level results in intracellular hyperglycemia that damages cells by the following mechanisms [27]: (1) increased activity of the aldose reductase/sorbitol pathway, (2) increased production of advanced glycation end products (AGE), and (3) increased synthesis of diacylglycerol (DAG) with generation of protein kinase C (PKC). All these actions lead to overproduction of superoxide by the mito-chondrial electron transport chain, which reduces availability of NO [27]. In type 2 diabetes, there is an early endothelial injury, most probably due to hyperglycemia, hypertension, dyslipidemia, and insulin resistance. Impaired endothelial dysfunction is also observed in the early stages of diabetes, in impaired glucose toler-ance, and in first-degree relatives of type 2 diabetics. In endothelial dysfunction there is a loss of NO secretion, secretion of angiotensin-II (A-II), and endothelin. These substances mediate vasoconstriction, promote thrombosis, and activate platelets. They are proinflammatory, and in the absence of NO they induce growth of VSMCs and stimulate the adhesion molecules ICAM and VCAM.

Adipocytes contribute to endothelial dysfunction in several ways. They express inflammatory cytokines such as IL-6 and TNF-α, which affect hepatic CRP synthesis, which in turn has been shown to down-regulate eNOS in vitro. Adipose expression of TNF-α may have a direct effect on endothelial cells. Studies show that endothelial-dependent dysfunction occurs soon after a fatty meal, perhaps via a pro-oxidant effect of triglyceride-rich lipoproteins [68]. The severity of impairment has been linked to the magnitude of the postprandial triglyceride rise.

HYPERTENSION

Q: What is the link between insulin resistance and hypertension in the metabolic syndrome?
The issue of the relationship among high blood pressure, insulin resistance, and CVD is complicated. Although the suspicion of an interrelation between hypertension and insulin resistance has existed for a long time, it was DeFronzo and Ferrannini [69] who observed that patients with essential hypertension were insulin resistant as determined by the euglycemic hyperinsulinemic clamp; this observation focused attention on this component of the metabolic syndrome. However, when assessed by the concen-tration of fasting insulin, the homeostasis model assessment (HOMA), or the HOMA insulin resistance index (HOMA-IR) [3], insulin resistance contributes only moderately to the increased prevalence of hypertension in the metabolic syndrome.

Hypertension is strongly associated with obesity and com-monly occurs in insulin-resistant individuals. Some experts believe that hypertension is less metabolic than other metabolic syndrome components. There are several mechanisms that are responsible for the link between hypertension and insulin resistance:

1. Sodium retention due to the antinatriuretic properties of insulin: Acute elevation of plasma insulin can reduce sodium excretion, and thus lead to sodium retention. Insulin is a vasodilator and when given intravenously to people with normal weight, with secondary effects on sodium reabsorption in the kidneys [3]. Evidence shows that sodium reabsorption is increased in whites but not in Africans or Asians with the metabolic syndrome [3]. In the presence of insulin resistance, the vasodilatory effect of insulin can be lost, whereas the renal effect on sodium reabsorption is preserved.
2. Increased vascular tone caused by reduced bioavailability of NO because of increased oxidative stress [1].
3. Increased asymmetric dimethylarginine (ADMA) levels [1].
4. Increased expression of angiotensinogen by adipose tissue, resulting in activation of the rennin-angiotensin system.
5. Increased sympathetic tone [3].
6. Proliferation of vascular smooth muscle cells.
7. Fatty acids, which themselves can mediate relative vasoconstriction.

Insulin also increases the activity of the sympathetic nervous system, an effect that may also be preserved in the presence of insulin resistance [3]. Supraphysiological levels of insulin stimulate the sympathetic nervous system in normal individuals in a dose-dependent manner. It has been proposed that hyperinsulinemia can lead to chronic increased sympathetic nervous system activity, and thereby increase sodium retention, peripheral vascular resistance, and cardiac output, subsequently raising the blood pressure. Despite this, little is known about the relationship of hypertension to other components of the metabolic syndrome and its relationship to insulin resistance and hyperinsulinemia.

Some authorities have suggested that hypertension can cause insulin resistance, rather than the reverse. This could be the result of closure of small vessels by capillary hypertrophy, leading to reduced blood flow, impairing the delivery of insulin to the local muscle bed. Fatty acids themselves can mediate relative vasoconstriction.

A study showed that blood pressure is significantly correlated with insulin resistance in normal-weight Caucasians. However, no significant correlation between blood pressures and insulin resistance is observed in most studies involving obese individuals or in many races other than Caucasians [70].

Patients with hypertension are glucose intolerant and hyper-insulinemic when compared with a matched group of individuals with normal blood pressure; as many as 50% of an unselected population with hypertension may show these changes [71]. The presence of hyperinsulinemia and glucose intolerance in a patient with high blood pressure indicates that resistance to insulin-stimulated glucose uptake also may be present. As with hyperinsulinemia, the defect in insulin action is present in both obese and nonobese individuals with hypertension and still can be detected after the blood pressure is well controlled with pharmaceutical agents [72].

The fact that insulin resistance and hyperinsulinemia both are present in individuals with hypertension raises the possibility that these changes may play a role in regulation of blood pressure. For instance, hyperinsulinemia has been shown both to enhance renal sodium retention and to enhance sympathetic nervous system activity; these actions lead to elevated blood pressure [72]. Another observation that supports the idea that changes in insulin metabolism may modulate blood pressure is that as many as 50% of patients with essential hypertension appear to be insulin resistant and hyperinsulinemic.

Additionally, abnormalities of insulin metabolism can be observed in normotensive first-degree relatives with high blood pressure [73] but not in individuals with secondary forms of hypertension [74].

However, the following three findings explain how insulin resistance and hyperinsulinemia are linked to essential hypertension. First, hypertensive patients as a group are insulin resistant and hyperinsulinemic. Second, normotensive first-degree relatives of individuals with essential hypertension are more insulin resistant. Third, hyperinsulinemia as a surrogate estimate of insulin resistance has been shown to predict subsequent development of essential hypertension [75]. Although only half of hypertensive patients are noted to be insulin resistant, those hypertensive patients who have other components of the metabolic syndrome are at increased risk of development of CVD. The Copenhagen Male Study [76] found that CVD risk was not increased in individuals with hypertension in the absence of elevated triacylglycerol and low HDL-C levels. On the contrary, the individuals with high blood pressure who had high triacylglycerol and low HDL cholesterol levels were at greater risk. This finding supports the concept that the association of hypertension with other components of the metabolic syndrome can be attributed to the concomitant existence of insulin resistance and hypertension.

Insulin resistance plays a crucial role in hypertension and atherosclerosis, and it is present to some extent in most hypertensive individuals. Approximately 50% hypertensive individuals are hyperinsulinemic, and up to 75% of people with type 2 diabetes are hypertensive. Abnormal glucose metabolism is seen in about two-thirds of patients presenting with an acute coronary syndrome (with about equal numbers of patients having impaired fasting glucose and overt disease) [1].

Two views reject the involvement of insulin resistance and hyperinsulinemia in the causation of hypertension. First, acute hyperinsulinemia in humans leads to vasodilation, and consequently blood pressure does not rise. Additionally, blood pressure falls when the insulin dose is reduced in obese hypertensive patients with NIDDM, and blood pressure increases when insulin treatment is started in patients with NIDDM that was poorly controlled by oral antidiabetic drugs. It has been suggested that the relationship between insulin level and blood pressure cannot always be observed in population studies [77]. Second, the study of racial differences in the relationship between blood pressure and insulin resistance [78] showed that blood pressure and insulin concentration were significantly correlated in whites but not in blacks or Pima Indians. However, blacks with hypertension are insulin resistant and hyperinsulinemic when compared with blacks with normal blood pressure [79], raising doubts on the significant role of insulin resistance in hypertension.

Increased circulating methylarginine (MA) has been linked to the metabolic syndrome to explain endothelial dysfunction and CVD risk. Proteins that contain MA are regulatory and they release it during catabolism. It has been suggested that increased protein turnover in insulin-resistant states contributes to an increase in circulating MA [80]. This study noted that obesity, sex, and aging have an effect on MA. Elevation of three MAs (asymmetrical dismethylarginine [ADMA], symmetrical dismethylarginine [SDMA], and N-monomethyl-L-arginine [NMMA] in the obese) and of ADMA in elderly men is related to increased protein turnover and to lesser insulin sensitivity of protein metabolism endothelial dysfunction. Asymmetric dimethylarginine is elevated in patients with type 2 diabetes. A glucose-induced impairment of dimethylaminohydrolase causes ADMA accumulation, and may contribute to endothelial vasodilator dysfunction in diabetes mellitus.

GLUCOSE INTOLERANCE

Q: What is the link between glucose intolerance and insulin resistance?
Impaired glucose tolerance (IGT) is a stage of impaired glucose regulation that lies between the normal range and the level

considered diagnostic of diabetes. The prevalence of IGT varies widely, being 3% to 10% in European populations and about 17% among overweight Americans. It is much higher in Asian Indians, Native Americans, Pacific Islanders, and indigenous Australians. There are an estimated 300 million people who have IGT worldwide [81]. Prediabetes includes IFG and IGT. About 70% to 75% of individuals with prediabetes meet the clinical criteria of the metabolic syndrome. Prediabetes carries a predictive power of CVD similar to that of the metabolic syndrome. But this predictive potential most likely can be explained by accompanying metabolic risk factors [82]. About 75% of individuals with prediabetes and 86% of individuals with type 2 diabetes have the metabolic syndrome. In 2003, the American Diabetes Association (ADA) reduced the level of IFG to 100–125 mg/dL (5.6 to 6.9 mmol/L). With this change, the prevalence of IFG increased about threefold from 7% to 24% in the U.S. in the NHANES study [81]. This was similar in all ethnic groups, but the increase was more pronounced in the younger age group of 20 to 50 years (almost fivefold) than in the age group $\geq$ 65 years (2.5-fold increase). With these new criteria, worldwide 30% to 40% of the adult population is considered to have IFG in contrast to 7% to 10% with the old criteria (Table 2.5).

Both IGT and IFG are associated with an approximately equal risk of diabetes. Those individual who have both IGT and IFG have even higher risk. There is dearth of evidence in the prevention of diabetes in patients with IFG. Annual progression from prediabetes to diabetes is about 10%, and some revert to normal. Impaired glucose tolerance is more common in women, whereas IFG is more common in men. The lifetime risk of developing diabetes is estimated at about 32.8% for men and 38.5% for women born in the U.S. in the year 2000 [83]. However, those who have one or more components of the metabolic syndrome are more likely to progress to diabetes. Prediabetes carries a predictive power of ASCVD, similar to that of metabolic syndrome. A test of IGT (2 hours postglucose) seems to be a better predictor of CVD and mortality than does the fasting glucose level. However, not all studies support the idea that lowering fasting glucose from 6.1 mmol/L (110 mg/dL) to 5.6 mmol/L (100 mg/dL) decrease CVD mortality [84]. Several conditions encountered in clinical practice confer an increased risk of type 2 diabetes. These include IFG, IGT, obesity, gestational diabetes, hypertension, hyperlipidemia, and menopause. It is interesting that the studies show that type 2 diabetes is preventable (at least to some extent) even among those at highest risk.

TABLE 2.5. Diagnostic criteria of diabetes mellitus

		Capillary whole blood	Venous plasma
Fasting glucose or 2 hours postglucose or random blood glucose with symptoms of diabetes; values proposed	DM	≥110 mg/dL/ ≥6.1 mmol/L ≥200 mg/dL/ ≥11.1 mmol/L	≥126 mg/dL/ ≥7.0 mmol/L ≥200 mg/dL/ 11.1 mmol/L
Fasting glucose	IGT	<110 mg/dL/ <6.1 mmol/L	<126 mg/dL/ <7.0 mmol/L
2 hours postglucose		140–199 mg/dL/ 6.8–11.0 mmol/L	140–199 mg/dL/ 7.8–11.0 mmol/L
Fasting glucose	IFG	NA*	100–125 mg/dL/ 5.6–6.9 mmol/L[a]
2 hours post glucose*		<140 mg/dL/ <7.8 mmol/L[b] <200 mg/dL/ <11.1 mmol/L[c]	<140 mg/dL/ <7.8 mmol/L[b] <200 mg/dL/ 11.1 mmol/L[c]

DM, diabetes mellitus; IFG, impaired fasting glucose; IGT, impaired glucose tolerance.
*If measured; no equivalent capillary whole blood.
[a]According to ADA (2003).
[b]WHO (1999).
[c]ADA (1997).
To convert glucose level in mmol/L into mg/dL, multiply by 18.
To convert plasma glucose from mg/dL to mmol/L multiply by 0.0555.

Epidemiological studies demonstrate that although both IFG and IGT represent an intermediary state between IGT and overt diabetes, they define two distinct populations with only partial overlap. Over half of IFG individuals have a 2-hour glucose <7.8 mmol/L and only 20% to 25% of individuals have a fasting plasma glucose >6.1 mmol/L [85].

The prevalence of IFG and IGT differs in various populations, but generally IFG has a lower prevalence than IGT. The condition also differs in their age and gender distribution. It has been suggested that although both conditions have underlying insulin resistance, they differ in the site of insulin resistance. Those with IFG predominantly have hepatic insulin resistance and normal muscle insulin sensitivity, whereas those with IGT have normal to slightly reduced hepatic insulin sensitivity and moderate to severe muscle insulin resistance [85].

The pattern of impaired insulin secretion also differs between IFG and IGT. Those individuals with isolated IFG have a decrease in the early-phase insulin response, but a late-phase insulin response during an oral glucose tolerance test (OGTT) is less severely impaired than in IGT. This is in contrast to IGT, which manifests severe defects in both early- and late-phase insulin responses. These insights provide some guidance as to the best route to follow in preventing progression from IFG and IGT to overt diabetes. Those individuals with IFG are more likely to benefit from agents targeting hepatic insulin resistance (e.g., metformin), whereas those with IGT are more likely to respond to agents targeting skeletal muscle insulin resistance (i.e., TZDs).

The defect in insulin action on glucose metabolism causes deficiencies in its ability to suppress glucose production by the liver and kidney and mediate glucose uptake and metabolism in insulin-sensitive tissues such as muscles and adipose tissue. The relationship among IFG, IGT, and insulin resistance is well accepted [3]. Hyperinsulinemia results in an effort to sustain euglycemia. The insulin resistance of islet β cells means that signals that generate glucose-dependent insulin secretion are malfunctioning, which is likely due to FFAs. Experimental elevation of FFAs affects both insulin action and insulin secretion. Prolonged exposure to elevated concentrations of FFAs contributes directly to the deterioration of β-cell function that accompanies the development of diabetes [86]. This results mainly due to lipotoxicity, though there are several mechanisms [3]. Insulin can also feed back on its own secretion. When the insulin receptor is deleted in skeletal muscle, hyperglycemia does not occur [3]. However the β-cell–specific knockout of the insulin receptor produces progressive glucose intolerance and diabetes [3]. In people with a genetic predisposition for diabetes, the presumed stress of an insulin-resistant environment on β cells causes glucose intolerance and subsequently diabetes [3]. There is a dynamic relationship between insulin resistance and compensatory insulin in β-cell mass and β-cell glucose metabolism. When a compensatory relationship is satisfactory, a normal glucose level is maintained. However, when β-cell compensation falls, the glucose level rises, leading to IGT or overt diabetes. Individuals who develop type 2 diabetes have a complex phenotype, with defects in insulin secretion, increased hepatic glucose production, and resistance to the action of insulin, all of which contribute to overt hyperglycemia. An increase in insulin, FFA or glucose levels may increase ROS generation and oxidative stress, as well as activate stress-sensitive pathways. This can further deteriorate both insulin action and secretion, thereby accelerating the progression to overt type 2 diabetes.

Impaired glucose tolerance is a risk factor for increases in cardiovascular mortality [87]. Many individuals with normal fasting glucose levels have insulin resistance. A recent application of the ATP-III, metabolic syndrome criteria to individuals in the NHANES study showed that impaired glucose criteria were only met in 10% of metabolic syndrome subjects, consistent with a significant underestimation of insulin resistance using this approach [81]. Impaired fasting glucose (100 to 125 mg/L) usually is an indicator of insulin resistance and is frequently accompanied by other metabolic factors; measurement of fasting glucose in overweight and obese patients is a reasonable option. If an OGTT is done, some individuals with IFG may be found to have IGT or even diabetes. Therefore, the WHO has recommended that these individuals should have an OGTT, if possible. Like IGT, IFG also has a high risk of progressing to type 2 diabetes.

CHRONIC KIDNEY DISEASE (MICROALBUMINURIA)

Q: What components of the metabolic syndrome are likely to be associated with chronic kidney disease?

Chronic kidney disease (CKD) is a long-term, often progressive loss of normal kidney function. It frequently leads to CVD and other complications related to end-stage kidney failure. In the United Kingdom, CKD affects 10% of the population and is often asymptomatic until renal function is severely reduced. Estimated glomerular filtration rate (eGFR) is an early marker of kidney disease. It is normally 100 mL/min, so the result roughly indicates the percentage of normal kidney function; that is, an eGFR of 45 mL/min means kidney function is about 40% of normal. The following are the five stages of CKD: stages 1 (GFR ≥90) and 2 (GFR 60–89), with normal or mildly reduced glomerular filtration rate (GFR); stage 3, moderate, GFR of 30 to 59 mL/min; stage 4, severe, GFR of 15 to 29 mL/min, stage 5, end stage, GFR <15 mL/min.

Chronic kidney disease has become an important public health challenge in the United States. According to data from the NHANES-III, 8.3 million (4.6%) of U.S. adults, 20 years of age or older, have CKD [88]. Chronic kidney disease is a major risk factor for end-stage renal disease, cardiovascular disease, and premature death [88]. Epidemiological studies have demonstrated that diabetes and hypertension are major risk factors for the development and progression of CKD and microalbuminuria. Chronic kidney disease is defined as a GFR of less than 60 mL/min per 1.73 m^3, and microalbuminuria is defined as a urinary albumin/creatinine ratio of 30 to 300 mg/g, and clinical proteinuria as urinary/creatine ratio greater than 300 mg/g. There are sparse data on the relationship between the metabolic syndrome and risk of chronic kidney disease [89]. Chen et al [90] detected a strong, positive, and significant relationship between the metabolic syndrome and the risk for CKD and microalbuminuria. Microalbuminuria has been shown to be a risk factor for the development of diabetic nephropathy and for macrovascular disease in both diabetics and nondiabetics.

Several studies have noted the association between insulin resistance and risk of CKD. Hoehner and colleagues [89] observed that individuals with three or more traits for the insulin resistance syndrome (hypertension, IFG, high fasting insulin level, high triglycerides, and low HDL) had 2.3-fold higher odds of microalbuminuria than individuals with no traits. Microalbuminuria is associated with insulin resistance in nondiabetics. In logistic regression analysis a weak relationship was observed between increasing insulin sensitivity and a decreasing prevalence of microalbuminuria. The relationship was partially dependent on blood pressure, plasma glucose level, and obesity. However, the mechanism by which insulin resistance and hyperinsulinemia produce microalbuminuria is not clearly understood.

The risk of CKD and microalbuminuria increased progressively with a higher number of components of the metabolic syndrome. These relationships were independent of age, sex, race, or ethnicity, or other potential risk factors for CKD, such as nonsteroidal anti-inflammatory drug (NSAID) use, education, physical inactivity, and cigarette smoking [81]. It is well understood that diabetes and hypertension are the major risk factors for the development and progression of CKD and microalbuminuria. However, few epidemiological studies have found that a reduced HDL cholesterol or elevated triglycerides relate to an increased risk for CKD. In a community study, high triglycerides and low HDL cholesterol predicted an increased risk for renal dysfunction [88]. Chen et al showed additional evidence that low HDL cholesterol and elevated triglyceride levels are associated with an increased risk of CKD and microalbuminuria. This study also showed that abdominal obesity is associated with a twofold increase in the odds of chronic renal disease. A meta-analysis showed that lipid lowering preserves GFR and decreases proteinuria in renal disease [88].

SMOKING

Q: Is there evidence that smoking predisposes to the metabolic syndrome?

Weitzman et al [91] demonstrated a dose-response, cotinine-confirmed relationship between tobacco smoke and the metabolic syndrome among adolescents in the U.S. The findings indicated that exposure to tobacco smoke, whether by active smoking or exposure to environmental tobacco smoke (ETS), is associated with at least a fourfold increase in the risk of the metabolic syndrome among adolescents who are overweight or at risk for becoming overweight. The mechanism underlying this increased risk of the metabolic syndrome is not clear. However, it has been suggested that a complex interaction involving insulin resistance is modified by social, environmental, racial/ethnic, and genetic factors. Additionally, studies have shown that smoking is associated with increased insulin resistance in adults, and may cause a primary defect leading to endothelial dysfunction, abnormal lipid metabolism, and accelerated cardiovascular disease [92]. If this concept is correct, then smoking and ETS exposure may be causally related to insulin resistance, which in turn may cause, contribute to, or trigger the metabolic abnormalities in overweight individuals that lead to the metabolic syndrome. A growing body of evidence also indicates that tobacco is independently associated with insulin resistance, and that insulin resistance may contribute to the accelerated atherosclerosis [92]. Tobacco smoke is associated with dyslipidemia, endothelial dysfunction, and a hypercoagulable state, all of which are components of metabolic syndrome.

PHYSICAL INACTIVITY

Q: What are the effects of physical activity vs. physical inactivity on the metabolic syndrome?

Approximately 70% of the U.S. population is classified as being sedentary. Physical inactivity is a major underlying risk factor for CHD. It enhances the lipid and nonlipid risk factors of the metabolic syndrome. It may augment the risk by reducing cardiovascular fitness and coronary blood flow. Physical inactivity is associated with insulin resistance and subsequent diabetes. There is good evidence of its association with insulin resistance syndrome, which may have some genetic cause or entail very strong environmental factors [4].

Physical activity reduces VLDL cholesterol, raises HDL cholesterol, and in some individuals lowers LDL cholesterol. It is also able to reduce blood pressure, reduce insulin resistance, and favorably affect cardiovascular outcome. High levels of physical activity have quite consistently protected against the development of diabetes and cardiovascular disease, conditions that are commonly associated with the metabolic syndrome. Men with high cardiorespiratory fitness were nearly two-thirds less likely to develop the metabolic syndrome. Even a low level of leisure-time physical activity (LTPA) tended to decrease the likelihood of developing the metabolic syndrome.

Low cardiovascular fitness is associated with the development of the metabolic syndrome independently of obesity and other important confounding factors. Physical activity improves the insulin resistance syndrome and vascular problems [93]. Regular and sustained physical activity improves all risk factors of the metabolic syndrome [94]. More intense exercise taken more often and for longer periods reduces cardiovascular risk more than less intense exercise. Recreational physical activities, rather than employment-related activities, appear to lead more closely to weight change. A greater increase in physical activity has larger effects on body composition and cardiovascular fitness [4].

ADVANCING AGE

Q: What factors in aging contribute to insulin resistance?
The demographic factor that seems to contribute to insulin resistance is advancing age. Insulin resistance increases with age, independent of changes in total adiposity. Aging entails a progressive derangement of the individual's internal environment, which leads to increased mortality rates with advancing age [46]. The metabolic and structural breakdown appears to result from diverse causes such as oxidative stress and inflammation. Insulin resistance and obesity accelerate aging because they are states of oxidative stress and inflammation, which bring about a shortened life span [94]. An increased incidence of insulin resistance and type 2 diabetes has frequently been observed with both natural aging and the progeria syndrome [95]. Various distinctive features of aging that could predispose to insulin resistance are increased fat mass (particularly increased visceral adiposity), increased circulating levels of inflammatory proteins, and increased cellular accumulation of triglycerides [46].

Interestingly, an observation in the elderly is that chronic restriction of energy intake remarkably improves survival and prevents the development of insulin resistance [96]. The effect, however, is largely due to prevention of abdominal obesity [46]. It has been suggested that an age-based decline in mitochondrial function promotes insulin resistance in the elderly [97]. It has also been proposed that age-induced resistance to the effect of leptin on fat distribution and insulin action adds to the increased tissue lipid accumulation and insulin resistance [98]. However, leptin resistance during aging is independent of fat mass.

HYPERURICEMIA

Q: What components of metabolic syndrome are associated with hyperuricemia?

An increase in serum uric concentration is commonly seen in association with glucose intolerance, dyslipidemia, and hypertension [77]. Hyperuricemia appears to be a member of the cluster of abnormalities comprising syndrome X. A study demonstrated that a significant correlation existed between serum uric acid concentration and both insulin resistance and the plasma insulin response to an oral glucose challenge test [77]. Thus hyperuricemia appears to be a member of the cluster of abnormalities comprising syndrome X. Moreover, resistance to insulin-mediated glucose uptake and the plasma insulin response are inversely correlated with the urinary excretion of uric acid, which indicates that a link between insulin metabolism and hyperuricemia was due to renal handling of uric acid. Additionally, individuals with asymptomatic hyperuricemia have been observed to have higher plasma insulin responses to oral glucose, higher plasma triglycerides, lower HDL cholesterol levels, and higher blood pressure when compared with a well-matched group of volunteers [77].

OXIDATIVE STRESS

Q: What is oxidative stress and how is it related to insulin resistance and CVD?

Oxidative stress is a condition in which production of oxidants and free radicals exceeds the body's ability to inactivate them. The imbalance between ROS and cellular antioxidant defense systems may result from alteration of glucose metabolism or be secondary to activation or dysregulation of several enzymes not directly involved in glucose metabolism. Oxidative stress is thought to play a role in chronic inflammatory conditions such as development of atherosclerosis/CVD where the invasion of inflammatory mediators (monocytes and macrophages) in the plaque and release of reactive oxygen and nitrogen species are the prime incriminating components. Oxidation of LDL cholesterol is the key step in the development of atherosclerosis.

Vascular oxidative stress is associated with diabetes [46]. Diabetics also have a low level of glutathione but an increase in plasma extracellular superoxide dismutase, which is associated with retinopathy and nephropathy [46]. Oxidative stress exists in organs affected by diabetic complications. Prevention of oxidative stress prevents organ damage in animal models. Oxidative stress can cause cellular dysfunction by promoting formation of advanced glycation end products (AGEs), by inducing DNA strand breaks, and by activating poly (ADP-ribose) polymerase (PARP) by causing dysfunction of eNOS, and by activating p38 and other stress-activated pathways leading to apoptosis [46]. It has been suggested that activation of common stress-activated signaling pathway such as NF-κB, p38, MAPK, and NH_2-terminal jun kinases/stress-activated protein kinases by glucose and possibly FFAs leads to both insulin resistance and impaired insulin secretion [99]. Increased oxidative stress has been suggested as a unifying mechanism among many nutrient-activated pathways [100].

In the cell, elevated FFAs and hyperglycemia cause overproduction of superoxide at the mitochondrial port and NO overproduction through NOS. Protein kinase C (PKC) and NF-κB are also activated and promote overproduction of NADPH enzyme, which generates large amounts of superoxide. Excess production of NADPH and superoxide encourages formation of the strong oxidant peroxynitrate, which damages DNA [50]. DNA damage is a prerequisite for the activation of the nuclear enzyme poly (ADP-ribose) polymerase (DARP); this in turn reduces the glyceride-3-phosphate dehydrogenase (GAPDH) activity. This alteration leads to adipose and muscle tissue reduction of GLUT-4 dysfunction and subsequent insulin resistance in endothelial cells in endothelial dysfunction and impaired insulin secretion of β cells. This process may be prevented by pharmacotherapy, α-glucosidase inhibitor, calcium channel blockers, statins, ACE inhibitors, angiotensin receptor blockers (ARBs), and glitazones (TZDs) [50].

β-Cell Dysfunction and Oxidative Stress

As in muscle and fat cell, β cells are also prone to damage by excess calorie intake. β cells, like endothelial cells, are not dependent on insulin for glucose uptake. Hence, if excess calories are consumed, they cannot downregulate the influx of nutrients by means of insulin resistance, thus enabling intracellular concentrations to rise further.

Beta cells are especially sensitive to ROS; therefore, oxidative stress is more likely to cause damage to mitochondria and significantly blunt insulin secretion [101]. Moreover, it has been shown that oxidative stress produced by a short exposure of β-cell preparations to H_2O_2 increases production of p21 and decreases insulin in RNA, cytosolic ATP, and calcium flux in cytosol and mitochondria. The role of increased glucose metabolism in the causation of β-cell dysfunction is further substantiated by a study that showed that intracellular ROS increased 15 minutes after exposure to high glucose, and that this effect was blunted by inhibitors of mitochondrial function [102]. Impaired insulin secretion is associated with an FFA-induced increase in ROS. Both glucose and FFA can impair insulin secretion in β cells by activating uncoupling protein [103]. In hyperglycemia this activation is induced by hyperglycemia-induced superoxide formation in mitochondria [102]. Consequently, because glucose as well as FFA overload are present during increased calorie disposal, it is likely that the combination with high glucose will maximize β-cell toxicity.

References

1. Reaven GM. Banting Lecture. Role of insulin resistance in human disease. Diabetic 1988;37:1595–1607.
2. Grundy SM, Brewer HB, Cleeman JI, et al. Definition of metabolic syndrome. Circulation 2004;109:433–438.
3. Eckel RH, Grundy SM, Zimmet P. The metabolic syndrome. Lancet 2005;365:9468–9415.
4. Stanner S. Cardiovascular Disease: Diet, Nutrition and Emerging Risk Factors. British Nutrition Foundation. London: Blackwell, 2005.
5. Statnick MA, Beavers LS, Conner LJ, et al. Decreased expression of apMI in omental and subcutaneous adipose tissue in human with type 2 diabetes. Int J Exp Diabetes Res 2000;1:81–88.
6. Lewis GF, Carpentier A, Adeli K, et al. Disordered fat storage and mobilization in the pathogenesis of insulin resistance and type 2 diabetes. Endocr Rev 2002;23:201–229.
7. Virtanen KA, Lonnroth P, Parkkola R, et al. Glucose uptake and perfusion in subcutaneous and visceral adipose tissue during insulin stimulation in nonobese and obese humans. J Clin Endocrinol Metab 2002;87:3902–3910.
8. Goodpaster BH, Kelly DE, Wing RR,, et al. Effects of weight loss on regional fat distribution and insulin sensitivity in obese. Diabetes 1999;48:839–849.
9. Das UN. Metabolic syndrome X is common in South Asians, but why and how? Nutrition 2002;18:774–776.
10. Banerji MA, Faridi N, Atluri R, et al. Body composition, visceral fat, leptin and insulin resistance in Asian Indian men. J Clin Endocrinol Metab 1999;84:137–144.
11. Aruirre V, Uchida T, Yenush L, et al. The c-JUN NH_2–terminal kinase promoted insulin resistance during association with IRS-1 and phosphorylation of ser^{307}. J Biol Chem 2000;275:9047–9054.
12. Waeber G, Delplanque J, Bonny C, et al. The gene MAPK 81 PI, encoding islet brain-1 is a candidate for type 2 diabetes. Nat Genet 2000;24:291–295.
13. Kolovou GD, Anagnostopoulou KK, Cokkinos DV. Pathophysiology of dyslipidemia in the metabolic syndrome. Postgrad Med J 2005;81: 358–366.
14. Halle M, Berg A, Garwers U, et al. Influence of 4 week's intervention by exercise and diet on LDL subfractions in obese men with type 2 diabetes. Metabolism 1999;48:641–644.

15. Grundy SM, Cleeman JI, Daniels SR, et al. Diagnosis and management of the metabolic syndrome (AHA.NHLBI). Circulation 2005;112: 2735–2752.

16. Han TS, Sattar N, Williams K, et al. Prospective study of CRP in relation to the development of diabetes and metabolic in the Mexico City Diabetes Study. Diabetes Care 2002;25:2016–2021.

17. Festa A, D'Agustine RJ, Howard G, et al. Chronic subclinical inflammation as part of the insulin resistance syndrome. Circulation 2000; 102:42–47.

18. Ridker PM, Buring JE, Cook NR. CRP, the metabolic syndrome, and risk of incident CV events. Circulation 2003;107:391–397.

19. Ridker PM. Rosuvastatin in the primary prevention of CVD among patients with low levels of LDL-C and elevated hsCRP protein. Circulation 2003;108:2292–2297.

20. Rulter MK, Meigs JB, Sullivan LM, et al. CRP, the metabolic, and prediction of CV events in the Framingham Offspring Study. Circulation 2004;110:380–385.

21. Anand SS, Razak F, Yi Q, et al. CRP as a screening test for CV risk in the multiethnic population. Arterioscler Thromb Vasc Biol 2004; 24:1509–1515.

22. Ford ES, Giles WH, Myer GL, et al. CRP concentration distribution among US children and young adults. Clin Chem 2003;49:1353–1357.

23. Yudkin JS, Stehouwer CD, Emeis JJ, et al. CRP in healthy subjects association with obesity, insulin resistance and endothelial dysfunction. Arterioscler Thromb Vasc Biol 1999;19:972–978.

24. Hotamisligil GS, Shargill NS, Spiegelman BM. Adipose expression of TNF-α: direct role in obesity-inked insulin resistance. Science 1993; 259:87–91.

25. Beuter B, Cerami A. The biology of cachectin/TNF-α. Annu Rev Immunol 1989;7:625–655.

26. Hotamisligil GS, Arner P, Carol F, et al. Increased adipose tissue expression of TNF-α in human obesity and insulin resistance. J Clin Invest 1995;95:2409–2415.

27. Barnet AH, Sudhesh K. Obesity and Diabetes. New York: John Wiley, 2004:49-78, 167–199.

28. Zhang Y. Proenca R, Maffie M, et al Positional cloning of the mouse obese gene and its human homologue. Nature 1994;372:425–432.

29. Sweeney G. Leptin signaling. Cell Signal 2002;14:655–663.

30. Minokoshi Y, Kim YB, Perini OD, et al. Leptin stimulates protein kinase. Nature 2002;415:339–343.

31. Koc E, Ustundag G, Aliondioglu D, et al. J Pediar Endocrinal Metab 2003;16:1283–1287.

32. Zhang Y, Proenca R, Maffei M, Barone M, Leopold L, Friedman JM. Positional cloning of the mouse obese gene and its human homologue. Nature 1994;372:425–432.

33. Sorensen TIA, Echwald S, Holm J-C. Leptin in obesity. BMJ 1996;313:953–954.

34. Wallace AM, Mc Mohan AD, Packard CJ, et al. Plasma leptin and the risk of CVD in WOSCOPS. Circulation 2001;104:3052–3056.

35. Zimmet P, Boyko EJ, Collier GR, et al. Etiology of metabolic syndrome: potential risk of insulin resistance, and other players. Ann NY Acad Sci 1999;892:25–44.

36. Dandona P, Aljada A, Chaudhuri A, et al. Metabolic syndrome. A comprehensive perspective based on interactions between obesity, diabetes, and inflammation. Circulation 2005;111:1448–1454.

37. Sattar N, Wannamethee G, Sarwar N, et al. Adiponectin and CHD. Circulation 2006;114:623–629.

38. Boden G, Laakso M. Lipid and glucose in type 2 diabetes. Diabetes Care 2004;27:2253–2259.

39. Chandran M, Phillip SA, Ciaraldi T, et al. Adiponectin: more than another fat cell hormone? Diabetes Care 2003;26(8):2442–2450.

40. Diez JJ, Ilgesias P. The role of novel adipocyte-derived hormone adiponectin in human disease. Eur J Endocrinol 2003;148(3):293–300.

41. Combs TP, Rajvani UB, Berg AH, et al. A transgenic mouse with detection in the collagenous domain of adiponectin displays elevated circulating adiponectin and improved insulin sensitivity. Endocrinology 2004;145:(1);367–383.

42. Goldstein BJ, Sclia R. Adiponectin: a novel adipokine linking adipocytes and vascular function. J Clin Endocrinol Metab 2004;89:2563–2568.

43. Steppan CM, Bailey ST, Bhat S, et al. The hormone resistin links obesity to diabetes. Nature 2001;409:307–312.

44. Ciamflone K, Xia Z, Cheu LY. Critical review of acylation stimulation protein physiology in humans and rodents. Brochim Biophys Acta 2003;1609:127–143.

45. Sartipy P, Loskutoff D, Monocyte chemoattractant protein-1 in obesity and insulin resistance. Proc Natl Acad Sci USA 2003;100:7265–7270.

46. Khan CR, Weir GC, King GL. Joslin's Diabetes Mellitus. Philadelphia: Lippincott Williams & Wilkins, 2005:207–266, 425–448, 823–837.

47. Cook KS, Min HY, Johnson D,, et al. Adipsin: a circulating serine protease homolog secreted by adipose tissue and sciatic nerve. Science 1987;237:402-405.

48. Masuzaki H, Paterson J, Shinyama H, et al. A transgenic model of visceral obesity and metabolic syndrome. Science 2001;294:2166–2170.

49. Morton NM, Paterson JM, Masuzaki H, et al. Novel adipose tissue-mediated resistance to diet-induced visceral obesity in 11-β HSD-1 deficient mice. Diabetes 2004;53:931–938.

50. Byrne CD, Wild SH. The Metabolism Syndrome. New York: John Wiley, 2005:198–394.

51. Laaksonen DE, Niskanen L, Nyyssonen, et al. CRP and the development of the MS and diabetes in the middle aged men. Diabetologia 2004;47:1403–1410.

52. Fumeron F, Aubert R, Siddiq A, et al. Adiponectin gene polymorphism and adiponectin levels are independently associated with development of hyperglycemia during a 3-year period. Diabetes 2004;53:1150–1157.

53. Savage DB, Petersen KF, Shulman GI. Mechanisms of insulin resistance in humans and possible links with inflammation. Hypertension 2005;45:828–837.

54. Hirosumi J, Tuncman G, Hotamisligil GS, et al. A central role for JNK in obesity and insulin resistance. Nature 2002;420:333–336.

55. Yuan M, Konstantopoulos N, Lee J, et al. Reversal of obesity- and diet-induced insulin resistance with salicylates or targeted disruption of IKK-β. Science 2001;293:1673–1677.

56. Ueki K, Kondo T, Kahn CR. SOCS-1 and SOCS-3 cause insulin resistance through inhibition of tyrosine phosphorylation of insulin receptor substrate proteins by discrete mechanism. Mol Cell Biol 2004;24:5434–5446.

57. Cho H, Mu J, Kim JK, et al. Insulin resistance and a diabetes mellitus-like syndrome in mice lacking the protein kinase Ak2. Science 2001;292:1728–1731.

58. Mahanty P, Hamounda W, Garg P, et al. Glucose challenge stimulates ROS generation by leukocytes. J Clin Endocrinol Metab 2000;85:2970–2973.

59. Devraj S, Jailal I. LDL post secretary modification function, and CAM in type 2 diabetic patient with and without tocopherol supplementation. Circulation 2000;102:191–196.

60. Mohanty P, Ghanim H, Hamouda W, et al. Both lipid and protein intakes stimulate increased generation of reactive oxygen species by polymorphonuclear leukocytes and mononuclear cells. Am J Clin Nutr 2002;75:767–772.

61. Aljada A, Mohanty P, Ghanim H, et al. Increase in intranuclear nuclear factor kappaB and decrease in inhibitor kappaB in mononuclear cells after a mixed meal: evidence for a proinflammatory effect. Am J Clin Nutr 2004;79:682–690.

62. Dandona P, Mohanty P, Ghanim H, et al. The suppressive effect of dietary restriction and weight loss in the obese on the generation of reactive oxygen species by leukocytes, lipid peroxidation, and protein carbonylation. J Clin Endocrinol Metab 2001;86:355–363.

63. Dandona P, Mohanty P, Ghanim H, et al. Inhibitory effect of a two day fast on ROS generation by leucocytes and plasma ortho- tyrosine and meta-tyrosine concentrations. J Clin Endocrinol Metab 2001;86:2899–2902.

64. Wolever TMS. Dietary carbohydrates and insulin resistance in humans. Br J Nutr 2000;83:s97–s102.

65. Lovejoy JC. Dietary fatty acids insulin resistance. Curr Atheroscler Rep 1999;1:215–220.

66. Festa A, D'Agostino R, Leena M Jr, et al. Relative contribution of insulin and its precursors to fibrinogen and PAI-1 in a large population with different states of glucose tolerance. Atheroscler Thromb Vasc Biol 1999;19:262–268.

67. Mansfield M, Heywood D, Grant P. Circulatory levels of factor V11, fibrinogen and von Willebrand factor and features of insulin resistance in first degree relatives of patients with NIDDM. Circulation 1996;94:2171–2176.

68. Vogel RA, Corretti MC, Plotnick GD. Effects of a single high-fat meal on endothelial function in healthy subjects. Am J Cardiol 1997;79:350–354.

69. DeFronzo RA, Ferrannini E. Insulin resistance: a multifaceted syndrome responsible for NIDDM, obesity, hypertension, dyslipidemia, and ASCVD. Diabetic Care 1991;14:173–174.

70. Wass JAH, Shalet SM, Gale EAM. Oxford Textbook of Endocrinology, 1st ed. Oxford: Oxford University Press, 2002:1834–1839.

71. Zavoroni IS, Mazza E, Dall'aglio P, et al. Prevalence of hyperinsulinaemia in patients with high blood pressure. J Intern Med 1992;231:235–240.

72. Reaven GM. Insulin resistance, hyperinsulinaemia, hypertriglyceridemia, and hypertension: parallels between human disease and rodent models. Diabetes Care 1991;14:195–202.

73. Facchini F, Chen YDI, Clinkingbeard C, et al. Insulin resistance, hyperinsulinemia, and dyslipidemia in nonobese individuals with a family history of hypertension. Am J Hypertens 1992;5:694–699.

74. Shamiss A, Carroll J, Rosenthal T. Insulin resistance in secondary hypertension. Am J Hypertens 1992;5:26–28.

75. Taittonen L, Uhari M, Nuutinen M, et al. Insulin and blood pressure among healthy children. Am Hypertens 1996;9:193–199.

76. Jeppesen J, Hein HO, Suadicani P, et al. Low triglyceride-high density lipoprotein cholesterol and risk of ischemic heart disease. Arch Intern Med 2001;16:361–366.

77. Reaven GM. Pathophysiology of insulin resistance in human disease. Physiol Rev 1995;75:473–486.

78. Saad MS, Lillioja BL, Myomba C, et al. Racial differences in the relation between blood pressure and insulin resistance. N Engl J Med 1991;324:733–739.

79. Falkner B, Hulman S, Kushner H. Insulin-stimulated glucose utilization and borderline hypertension in young adult blacks. Hypertens Dallas 1993;22:18–25.

80. Marliss ED, Chevalier S, Gougeou R. Elevation of plasma methylarginines in obesity and ageing related to insulin sensitivity and rates of protein turnover. Diabetes 2006;49:351–359.

81. Ford ES, Giles WH, Deiltz WH. Prevalence of the metabolic syndrome among US adults: study of NHANES. JAMA 2002;287:356–359.

82. Haffner SM, Stern MP, Hazuda HP, et al. CV risk factors in confirmed prediabetes individuals. JAMA 1990;263:2893–2898.

83. Curtis J, Wilson C. Preventing type 2 diabetes mellitus. J Am Board Fam Pract 2005;18:37–43.

84. Sorkin JD, Muller DC, Fleg JL, et al. The relationship of fasting and 2–h post challenge plasma glucose concentration to mortality. Diabetes Care 2005;28:2626–2632.

85. Abdul-Ghani MA, Tripathy DD, DeFronzo RA. Contributions of beta-cell dysfunction and insulin resistance to the pathogenesis of IGT and IFG. Diabetes Care 2006;29(5):1130–1139.

86. Cavaghan MK, Ehrmann DA, Polonsky S. Interaction between insulin resistance and insulin secretion in the development of glucose intolerance. J Clin Invest 2000;106(3):329–333.

87. Ceriello A. The possible role of postprandial hyperglycemia in the pathogenesis of diabetic complications. Diabetologia 2003;46 (suppl 1):M9–M16.

88. Chen J, Muntner P, Hamm LL, et al. The metabolic syndrome and chronic kidney disease in US adults. Ann Intern Med 2004;140: 167–174.

89. Hoehner CM, Greenlund KD, Rith-Narjan S, et al. Association of insulin resistance syndrome and microalbuminuria among nondiabetic native Americans. J Am Soc Nephrol 2002;13:1626–1634.

90. Chen J, Munter P, Hamm LL, et al. Insulin resistance and risk of CKD in nondiabetic US adult. J Am Soc Nephrol 2003;14:469–477.

91. Weitzman M, Cook S, Auinger P, et al. Tobacco smoke exposure is associated with the metabolic syndrome in adolescence. Circulation 2005;112(6):862–864.

92. Facchini FS, Hollenbeck CB, Jeppesen J, et al. Insulin resistance and cigarette smoking. Lancet 1992;339:1128–1130.

93. Powell KE, Pratt M. Physical activity and health avoiding the short and miserable life. BMJ 1996;313:126–128.

94. Gardner J, Shengxn L, Sathanur S, et al. Rise in insulin resistance is associated with elevated telomere attention. Circulation 2005;111 (17):2171–2177.

95. Ferrannini E, Natali A, Capaldo B, et al. Insulin resistance, hyperinsulinaemia, and blood pressure: role of age and obesity: EGIR. Hypertension 1997;30:1144–1149.

96. Heilbronn LK, Ravussin E. Caloric restriction and aging. Am J Clin Nutr 2003;78:361–369.

97. Petersen KF, Befroy D, Dufour S, et al. Mitochondrial dysfunction in the elderly. Science 2003;300:1140–1142.

98. Ma XH, Muzumdar R, Yang XM, et al. Aging is associated with resistance to effects of leptin on fat distribution and insulin action. J Gerontol A Biol Sci Med Sci 2002;57:B225–231.

99. Evans JL, Goldfine ID, Maddux BA, et al. Oxidative stress and stress-activated signaling pathways. Endocr Rev 2002;23:599–622.

100. Nishikawa T, Edelstein D, Du XL, et al. Normalizing mitochondrial superoxide production blocks three pathways of hyperglycemic damage. Nature 2000;404:787–890.

101. Robertson RP, Harmon J, Tran PO, et al. Glucose toxicity in β-cells: type 2 diabetes, good radicals gone bad, and glutathione connection. Diabetes 2003;52:581–587.

102. Sakai K, Matsumato K, Mishikwa T, et al. Mitochondrial ROS reduce insulin secretion by pancreatic beta-cell. Biochem Biophys Res Commun 2003;300:216–222.

103. Krauss S, Zhang CY, Scorrano L, et al. Superoxide-mediated activation of uncoupling protein 2 causes pancreatic beta-cell dysfunction. J Clin Invest 2003;112:1831–1842.

Chapter 3
Pathogenesis of the
Metabolic Syndrome

THE ROLE OF GENES

Q: What role do genes play in the mechanism of the metabolic syndrome?

A powerful genetic basis for insulin resistance is supported by its high prevalence in certain populations, especially the Nauru Islanders of the Pacific, the Pima Indians in Arizona, and the urban Wanigela people in Papua New Guinea. Also, there is almost a 100% association of insulin resistance with the diagnosis of type 2 diabetes in monozygotic twins but only a 20% association in dizygotic twins [1]. Environmental and genetic factors lead to obesity and insulin resistance, which contribute to metabolic abnormalities. The final outcome is cardiovascular disease. Twin, adoption, and family studies have shown that both genetic and environmental factors are important, with a heritable estimate of 30% to 70%. The environmental contribution of insulin resistance to the metabolic syndrome is estimated to be approximately 50%.

The association of gene variants, insulin resistance, and dyslipidemia is complex and the evidence is inconsistent. However, gene variants, and particularly the interaction between these variants and the environment, have an important role in glucose and lipoprotein metabolism.

The cascade of impaired glucose and lipid metabolism in the metabolic syndrome is affected by gene variants (polymorphism, mutations) in genes regulating insulin action in different tissues. The thrifty genotype hypothesis implies that the evolutionary selection of genes that initially had favorable effects for energy storage are harmful in the setting of the modern environment of physical inactivity and an excess of caloric intake. These genes are involved in both glucose and lipid metabolism [2]. Genes primarily regulating lipid and lipoprotein level can secondarily lead to insulin resistance in all target tissues and finally to impaired glucose metabolism.

A common polymorphism in the plasma cell (PC-1) insulin receptor substrate 1 and 2 and peroxisome proliferation–activated receptor-γ2 *(PPAR-γ2)* genes have been linked to insulin resistance and dyslipidemia, but the results have not been consistent [2]. However, the Pro12Pro genotype of the *PPAR-γ2* gene has been consistently associated with insulin resistance and the risk of type 2 diabetes. The promoter polymorphism in the hepatic lipase gene, the SU Thr allele of fatty acids binding protein 2 gene, and genes related to low-density lipoprotein (LDL) particle size have been linked with lipid metabolism, but their association with insulin resistant is not consistent.

Monogenic Components of Metabolic Syndrome

The example of a monogenic metabolic gene is *PPAR-γ*. Mutations in the *PPARγ* gene that disrupt the function of protein cause severe insulin resistance, dyslipidemia, and hypertension [3]. It has also been shown that treating the *PPARγ* mutation carriers with thiazolidinediones (TZDs) improves insulin sensitivity [3]. Farooq and O'Rahilly [4] have described monogenic obesity and insulin resistance disorders such as maturity onset diabetes of the young (MODY); the hypertension disorders (e.g., Gordon syndrome, Liddle's syndrome); and some disorders resulting in dyslipidemia. A single DNA mutation in a single gene causes one of the traits of the metabolic syndrome. The features of the monogenic (mendelian) form are one gene per family but one to 10 genes in the population, onset at a young age, strict (mendelian) inheritance pattern, and low environmental risk. Simple gene mutations in the genes for the melanocortin 4 receptor (Mc4R), propiomelanocortin (POMC), leptin, and the leptin receptor have been associated with obesity and insulin resistance. Individuals with severe obesity due to a mutation in the leptin gene show dramatic reductions in fat mass and lipid and insulin concentrations when treated with recombinant leptin [5].

Polygenic Diseases

In the polygenic form, there are more than one gene (usually ten) per family but usually 100 genes are involved in the population. There is a statistically increased risk relative to general population, and the onset is in middle to old age. The genetic polymorphism of the glucocorticoids receptor (GR) has been described that alters glucocorticoid hormone action and is associated with features of the metabolic syndrome. Altered patterns of GR expression in skeletal muscle are associated with the metabolic syndrome [6]. Polymorphisms in the locus for adiponectin and 3q27 could affect the level of adiponectin. A study showed evidence of linkage with the metabolic syndrome [7]. There is some increased type 2 diabetes susceptibility.

Genes Known to Alter the Risk of the Metabolic Syndrome

Common gene variants known to alter cholesterol and triglyceride blood concentrations are *ApoE, ApoAV,* cholesteryl ester transferase protein *(CETD)*, hepatic lipase *(HL)*, and lipoprotein lipase *(LPL)*. The common variants in the apolipoprotein E (ApoE) $e^2/e^3/e^4$ gene are the most studied. This gene is known to affect the response to dietary changes that may affect cardiovascular risk. Carriers of the $ApoE_4$ variant appeared to be hyperresponders in a study carried out by Sarkkinen et al [8]. They reduced their total plasma cholesterol more than did carriers of the $ApoE_3$ and E_2 variants on a low-fat diet. They also increased their total cholesterol more on cholesterol supplementation, which indicates a genotype-specific susceptibility of cholesterol feeding. The carriers of the ApoE allele are especially prone to develop the hypertriglyceridemic effect of a high-sucrose diet. The $ApoE_4$ variant also leads to a susceptibility to an increased risk of cardiovascular disease (CVD). In one study the CVD risk was increased by 26% in $ApoE_4$ carriers as compared to $ApoE_3$ carriers, and there was no effect on $ApoE_2$ carriers [9]. Carriers of the $ApoE_2$ variant have a risk that is similar to that of homozygous $ApoE_3$ carriers, although they had lower LDL cholesterol. This may explain why the few $ApoE_2$ carriers develop hyperlipidemia type III.

Calpain 10

A recent meta-analysis found that variants in the calpain 10 gene alter the risk of type 2 diabetes [10]. Inhibition of calpain proteases can increase the insulin-secretory response in mouse pancreatic β cells, and calpain 10 is probably important in β-cell apoptosis. Studies support the idea that calpain 10 polymorphisms are associated with insulin resistance, and a correlation have been demonstrated between the calpain 10 gene type and responses to oral glucose load.

The Kir 6.2 and SUR Genes

The sulfonylurea receptor SUR-I and the inwardly rectifying potassium channel Kir 6.2 form the subunit of adenosine triphosphate (ATP)-sensitive potassium channels in the β cells of the pancreas. Variants of SUR and Kir 6.2 cause rare diabetes-related disorders and predispose to type 2 diabetes [6]. Mutations in Kir 6.2 can cause two extremes of the β-cell phenotype: (1) hypoglycemia of infancy, and (2) a common variant in the Kir 6.2 gene (called *KCNJ11*) predisposes to type 2 diabetes.

The HNFl Gene
Hepatocyte nuclear factor-1α (HNF-1α) is a transcription factor expressed in liver and β cells of the pancreas. A severe mutation of HNF-1α causes MODY, and its common variant predisposes to type 2 diabetes.

The HNF4 Gene
The severe mutations of the *HNF4* gene situated in the region of chromosome 20 can cause MODY. The variation of the *HNF4* gene is significantly associated with type 2 diabetes.

The *GEK* Gene
Glucokinase (GCK) is the glucose-sensing enzyme of β cell. Its severe mutations cause MODY. A common variant in the promoter of the *GCK* gene (expressed in the β cells), GCK-30, is linked with fasting glucose across several studies [11].

Q: How are gene variants, insulin resistance, and dyslipidemia interrelated?

Genes Variants Regulating Primary Insulin Sensitivity
Several genes regulate insulin action, including the genes regulating insulin receptor function (PC-1), early insulin signaling (insulin receptor substrate), and nuclear receptors (PPAR-γ2).

PC-1
The class II transmembrane glucoprotein PC-1 is a potential candidate gene for insulin resistance and type 2 diabetes because it inhibits insulin receptor tyrosine kinase activity [12]. The K121Q polymorphism in exon 4 of the *PC-1* gene has been associated with insulin resistance in hyperglycemia but its role in dyslipidemia is not well studied [12].

Insulin Receptor Substrates (IRS)
Insulin receptor substrate type 1 (IRS-1) is a major substrate for the insulin receptor and it modulates insulin signaling in skeletal muscle, adipose tissue, and the vasculature. Hence, it is very likely a candidate gene for insulin resistance and type 2 diabetes. The most common variant of the *IRS-1* gene is the Gly972Arg substitution, which leads to an impairment in IRS-1–associated phosphatidylinositol (PI)-3-kinase activity [12]. Reduced insulin

sensitivity is observed in carriers of the Gly972Arg variant compared to carriers of the common genotype. Additionally, carriers of this polymorphism had many components of the metabolic syndrome such as raised triglycerides, total cholesterol/high-density lipoprotein (HDL) cholesterol ratio, free fatty acid (FFA) levels, systolic blood pressure, and intima media thickness [12]. This finding supports the idea that carriers of Gly972Arg substitution have a significantly increased body mass index (BMI), fasting insulin level, insulin resistance, and triglyceride level than do obese noncarriers [12]. Therefore, the Gly972Arg polymorphism in the *IRS-1* gene is likely associated with insulin resistance and dyslipidemia, which are components of the metabolic syndrome.

PPAR-γ2

Loss-of-function mutations cause lipodystrophy, and gain-of-function mutations lead to increased body mass. Laakso [12] found that the Pro12Ala substitution is associated with low body weight and BMI, high insulin sensitivity, a high HDL cholesterol level, and a low total triglyceride level. The Pro12Pro genotype is associated with type 2 diabetes. The Pro12Ala polymorphism of the *PPAR-γ2* gene regulates conversion to type 2 diabetes. In individuals born with a low birth weight, the Pro12Pro genotype was associated with increased insulin resistance and raised insulin level. The association between a common amino acid changing polymorphism (Pro12Ala in the *PPARγ* gene and type 2 diabetes was confirmed in a recent study [13].

Gene Variants Regulating Primarily Dyslipidemia

The examples of gene variants regulating dyslipidemia include those regulating HDL cholesterol (hepatic lipase), fat absorption (fatty acid building protein-2), and LDL particle size (cholesteryl ester transfer protein [CETP], lipoprotein lipase [LPL]).

Hepatic Lipase

Hepatic lipase is an important enzyme regulating the HDL cholesterol level through its activity of hydrolysis of triglycerides and phospholipids on plasma proteins. Gene–nutrient interactions affecting HDL cholesterol may contribute to individual variability in coronary heart disease (CHD) associated with dietary fat intake. The C514T polymorphism of the hepatic lipase gene seems to play an important role.

Fatty Acid Binding Protein (FABP) Type 2

The intestinal fatty acid binding protein (FABP) type 2 gene is expressed only in absorptive columnar epithelial cells of small intestine. It transports hydrophilic fatty acids from the plasma membrane to the endoplasmic reticulum, where FFAs are esterified to form triglycerides. The common polymorphism, Ala54Thr (only in Pima Indians) has been observed in the *FABP-2* gene, which could potentially associate with insulin resistance because raised dietary fat absorption causes high circulatory FFAs and triglyceride levels. This leads to impaired insulin action in skeletal muscle and increased gluconeogenesis in the liver [12]. It is probable that dietary factors could modify the lipoproteins as well as insulin action, supporting the possibility that a variant of the *FABP-2* gene may also have a gene-nutrient interaction [12].

Gene Variants Regulating Low-Density Lipoprotein Particle Size

Gene variants regulating LDL particle size can lead to insulin resistance and an increases risk of type 2 diabetes. CETD-629A and LPL 447X alleles were found to be associated with a moderately increased peaks particle size [12], whereas the lipoprotein E e⁴ allele was associated with marked reduction in LDL peak particle size and an increased relative proportion and plasma level of small, dense LDL. It was also noted that the interaction between the HL-480 C/T carrier and ApoE polymorphism plays a crucial role in the increased concentration of small, dense LDL in HL-280T carriers [12].

Lipodystrophy

Lipodystrophy is a group of disorders that are characterized by severe insulin resistance and partial or complete absence of adipose tissue. The study of these genetic disorders is important in understanding the mechanism of fat distribution and insulin resistance. In some instances, there is a potential interaction between separate genes in conferring an increased risk of insulin resistance. The combined effect of PC-1 and PPAR-γ2 polymorphisms results in significant increases in BMI and insulin levels and impairment in both insulin sensitivity and insulin secretion. In partial or complete lipoatrophy, insulin resistance and the metabolic syndrome typically coexist [14]. Evidence from the study of these diseases supports a genetic basis of the metabolic syndrome, including single gene defects in *PPARγ*, lamin A/C, 1-acyglycerol-3-phosphate, O-acyltransferase, seipin, β₂-adrenergic receptor, and adiponectin [14]. The mutations, polymorphisms, and syndromes (due to mutations in insulin receptor) are the following [15]:

1. Leprechaunism: the most extreme form associated with intrauterine growth retardation and characteristic dimorphic features (e.g., prominent eyes, thick lips, upturned nostrils, low-set

posteriorly rotated ears, thick skin, and lack of subcutaneous fat). Life expectancy is up to 1 year.
2. Rabson-Mendenhall syndrome: dimorphic features with premature or dysplastic teeth, gingivitis, and growth retardation. Life expectancy up to 15 years.
3. Type A insulin resistance: mildest; entails a characteristic triad of acanthosis nigricans, insulin resistance, and hyperandrogenism.
4. G972 R polymorphism of IRS-1.
5. Pseudoacromegaly: severe insulin resistance, acromegaly, and growth hormone normal.
6. M3261 polymorphism of p85.
7. Plasma–cell differentiation factor–1 (PC-1) polymorphism.
8. P115Q mutation of *PPARγ*: features of severe insulin resistance, and partial lipodystrophy of limbs.
9. Familial partial lipodystrophy (lamin A/C mutations).

Q: What is the pathophysiology of the metabolic syndrome?

Opinions differ as to whether the metabolic syndrome should be defined mainly by insulin resistance, by the metabolic consequences of obesity, by the risk of CVD, or simply by a collection of statistically related factors. In the pathogenesis of the metabolic syndrome, three important factors underline the process: (1) obesity and disorders of obese tissue, (2) insulin resistance, and (3) a constellation of independent factors (e.g., molecules of hepatic, vascular, and immunologic origin) that mediate specific components of metabolic syndrome. Aging, the proinflammatory state, hormonal changes, and endothelial dysfunction also contribute. Most of these factors were discussed in Chapter 2. Some are further discussed here. Experts differ about whether obesity/hypertriglyceridemic waist or insulin resistance is more important in the pathogenesis of the metabolic syndrome; this issue is further complicated by the fact that obesity and insulin resistance are strongly interrelated. In addition to obesity and insulin resistance, each risk factor of the metabolic syndrome is subject to regulation through both genetic and acquired factors, which leads to variability in the expression of risk factors. Lipoprotein metabolism is immensely modulated by genetic factors. Hence, expression of dyslipidemia as a result of obesity or insulin resistance varies considerably.

The most accepted hypothesis for the pathophysiology of the metabolic syndrome is insulin resistance. Insulin resistance, hyperinsulinemia, and overproduction of FFAs/nonesterified fatty acids (NEFAs) are the key features. The major insulin-responsive tissues are the liver, skeletal muscle, and adipose tissue, but action on myocardium, smooth muscle, endothelium, and vasculature also plays an important role. It is difficult to substantiate a unifying mechanism involved in the pathogenesis of the metabolic syndrome, and it is possible that a variety of incriminating factors play a role, some as secondary consequences of a primary abnormality or of several primary abnormalities. It is well accepted that FFAs impair glucose metabolism in insulin-sensitive tissues, such as muscle and liver. There are multiple mechanisms for this action, but they may be initiated by a single method—that is, increased energy availability). It is also accepted that FFAs impair cellular glucose uptake. However, there is a difference of opinion regarding the inhibitory effect of FFAs on glucose oxidation that has been suggested (by Randle) to be responsible for FFA-mediated inhibition of glucose uptake [16]. Although insulin resistance is still defined on the basis of the effect of insulin on glucose metabolism, during the last decade there has been a shift from the traditional "glucocentric" view of diabetes to an increasingly accepted "lipocentric" viewpoint [17].

In the pathophysiology of the metabolic syndrome the abnormality of increased lipolysis (resulting in excessive production of NEFA) and triglyceride storage in insulin-sensitive tissues (i.e., adipose tissue, skeletal muscle, liver, and pancreas) are the early manifestations. The sequence of events may be as follows: A state of positive energy balance sets in, due to obesity or excessive calorie intake. This is followed by triglyceride accumulation in adipose tissue, leading to insulin resistance at that site, which results in the diversion of fat/energy substrates from adipose to nonadipose tissues. The consequence of this sequence is the development of insulin resistance in other insulin-sensitive extraadipose tissues. This leads to a complex series of metabolic abnormalities in various tissues. Within the vasculature, the changes are associated with an increase in cellular reactivity such as activation of the endothelial cell, platelet, and monocyte. This association contributes to the procoagulant and proinflammatory state vascular phenotype that probably precedes the development of atheromatous plaques. Expression of inflammatory cytokines from an expanded mass causes a proinflammatory and prothrombotic state. An elevated FFA concentration provides a stimulus and substrate for hepatic triglyceride synthesis and for very low density lipoprotein (VLDL) assembly and secretion, contributing to dyslipidemia. An increased NEFA concentration also potentially may interfere with glucose metabolism by reducing glucose uptake and oxidation. Insulin resistance may lead to impaired endothelial function. Altered cellular glucocorticoid hormone also contributes to insulin resistance. The role of various contributors is demonstrated in Figure 3.1.

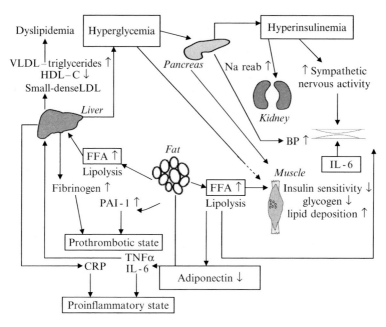

FIGURE 3.1. Pathophysiology of the metabolic syndrome. Reab, reabsorption. FFA, free fatty acid; HDL, high-density lipoprotein; LDL, low-density lipoprotein; PAI-1, plasminogen activator inhibitor-1; TNF-α, tumor necrosis factor-α; VLDL, very low density lipoprotein.

Pathophysiology of the Metabolic Syndrome

The pathophysiology of the metabolic syndrome entails the following:

- There is excessive release of FFAs from an enlarged adipose mass (increased lipolysis).
- FFAs act on liver to produce increased glucose, triglycerides (which reduces HDL cholesterol level), and VLDL.
- FFAs reduce insulin sensitivity in muscle by inhibiting insulin-mediated glucose uptake.
- Elevated plasma glucose (and possible elevated FFAs) increase pancreatic secretion, resulting in hyperinsulinism, which causes enhanced sodium reabsorption and increased sympathetic nervous system activity, leading to hypertension.
- Proinflammatory cells expressed by adipose tissue cause greater insulin resistance and lipolysis of triglyceride stores of adipose tissue.

- Elevated plasma tumor necrosis factor-α (TNF-α), interleukin-6 (IL-6), and other cytokines increase hepatic glucose production and enhance VLDL production of liver and insulin resistance in muscle.
- Elevated cytokines and FFAs also lead to overproduction of fibrinogen by liver and plasminogen activator inhibitor-1 (PAI-1) by adipose tissue, resulting in a prothrombotic state.
- Fatty acids lead to ectopic deposition of lipid in extraadipose tissue (e.g., muscle, liver, β cells), causing insulin resistance at these sites.
- Paracrine and endocrine effects of the proinflammatory state result in more secretion of TNF-α and IL-6, which accelerate insulin resistance and lipolysis of adipose tissue triglyceride stores to FFA; enhance hepatic glucose synthesis, VLDL expression, and insulin resistance in muscle; and increase fibrinogen and PAI-1 by the liver, causing a prothrombotic state.
- Reduced production of adiponectin by adipose tissue plays a role in the pathogenesis of the metabolic syndrome.

Q: What is the role of obesity in the development of the metabolic syndrome?

Obesity is associated with diminished insulin action and insulin resistance. There appears to be an inverse relationship between insulin sensitivity and visceral adiposity, independent of total adiposity (as measured by the BMI). There is a strong correlation between abdominal adiposity and type 2 diabetes, probably due to the increased metabolic activity of visceral adipocytes compared with subcutaneous depots. Insulin resistance in adipose tissue is characterized by decreased suppression of lipolysis in adipose tissue by insulin, leading to elevated FFAs. The quantity of FFAs from adipocytes that is released into the circulation corresponds to the size of the adipocytes and the overall fat mass of adipose tissue. The consequence of increased FFA lipolysis and reduced FFA fractional esterification in the metabolic syndrome and type 2 diabetes is diversion of FFAs toward nonadipose tissue such as liver, muscle, heart, and pancreatic β cells.

In visceral obesity, fatty acids derived from adipose tissue pass through the splanchnic circulation via the portal vein directly to the liver and thus affect glucose production, lipid synthesis, and secretion of prothrombotic proteins (i.e., fibrinogen and PAI-1). In the liver, NEFA is oxidized to acetyl coenzyme A (CoA), which stimulates pyruvate carboxylase, and hence gluconeogenesis production of glucose from pyruvate is increased (Fig. 3.2). Several factors such as increasing obesity, insulin resistance, visceral fat, other metabolic

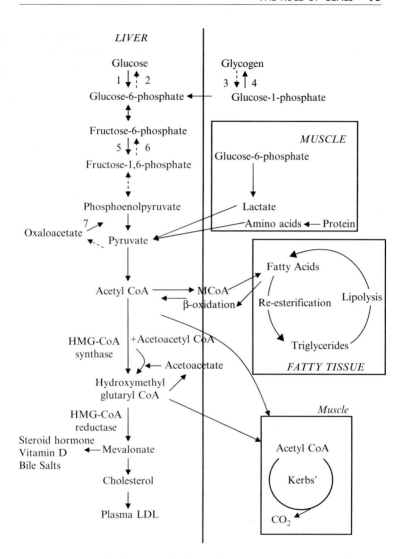

FIGURE 3.2. Carbohydrate metabolism. The important enzymes and steps that are affected by insulin are as follows: 1, glucokinase; 2, glucose-6-phosphatase; 3, phosphorylation; 4, glycogen dehydrogenase; 5, phospho-fructokinase; 6, fructose-1,6-biphosphatase; 7, phosphoenolpyruvate carboxykinase. HMG, hydroxymethylglutaryl; MCoA, malonyl-coenzyme A; →, increased action; ←----, decreased action.

factors, and increased lipolytic response to catecholamine result in enhanced lipolysis rate. This, along with venous drainage of intraperitoneal fat, exposes the liver to high levels of NEFAs and glycerol. This leads to excessive secretion of VLDL and triglycerides, resulting in hypertriglyceridemia.

In women, the increased postprandial FFAs released into the upper body obesity come from the nonsplanchnic upper body fat, and not from the visceral fat [18]. This indicates that visceral fat might be a marker for, but not the source of, excess postprandial fatty acids in obesity [18]. Abdominal subcutaneous fat, through lipolysis, releases products that pass into the systemic circulation directly and do not cause adverse effects through their effects on the liver.

Insulin resistance usually increases with increasing fat at any given level body fat. A BMI ≥30 invariably causes postprandial hyperinsulinemia and relatively low insulin sensitivity [19]. An inherited etiology also plays a role in insulin resistance, which is responsible for a spectrum of insulin sensitivities in an overweight person with a BMI ranging between 25 and 29.9. Among South Asian people, insulin resistance is known to occur at a much lower level of BMI (e.g., <25), which leads to a greater incidence of type 2 diabetes and increased cardiovascular risk in this population. Hence, their clinical management is stricter. *Primary insulin resistance* is the term used when insulin resistance occurs with only mild to moderate excess weight in this population. Asian Indians may even manifest excessive insulin resistance in the absence of obesity. Those with more inherent insulin resistance can develop the metabolic syndrome with only a moderate excess of abdominal fat, but some people with little or no inherent insulin resistance can develop the metabolic syndrome if they suffer from marked abdominal obesity.

Obesity is associated with insulin resistance, and the potential mechanism of this association is ectopic lipid accumulation. An inflammation response induces insulin resistance in two ways: First, activation of inflammatory signaling intermediates may be incriminated in serine phosphorylation of IRS-1 within insulin-sensitive tissues (e.g., hepatocytes and monocytes), thus inducing insulin resistance. This was discussed in Chapter 2. Second, inflammatory cell infiltration within adipose tissue may be responsible for altering the adipocyte lipid metabolism and cytokine production by adipose tissue, which has an adverse effect on metabolic important tissues.

Obesity may suppress insulin sensitivity through excess lipolysis caused by TNF-α. Obesity may act through release of abnormal amounts of various other products from adipose tissue, notably cytokines, leptin, and adiponectin. The production of IL-6 and other cytokines is enhanced, and they increase hepatic glucose production, production of VLDL by the liver, and insulin resistance in muscle. Cytokines and FFAs also augment the production of fibrinogen and PAI-1 by the liver, which complements the overproduction of PAI-1 by adipose tissue. This leads to a prothrombotic state. The mature adipocytes have a specific size capacity for efficient glucose uptake, and therefore an increasing adiposity correlates with enlarged adipocytes and insulin resistance, which may affect systemic insulin resistance and triglycerides storage. Weight fluctuation (weight cycling) occurs both in obese and lean individuals. Various harmful effects seem to occur with weight fluctuation, including an increased risk of insulin resistance and type 2 diabetes and an increased risk of CVD. Visceral adipocytes are not only relatively resistant to the action of insulin, but also manifest increased sensitivity to the lipolytic effects of catecholamine. Adiponectin acts to improve insulin action, but it is released in a smaller amount in obesity.

It has also been noted that the suppressive effect of insulin on FFA level is impaired in obese insulin-resistant individuals and in type 2 diabetes. A similar defect in glucose-tolerant first-degree relatives of patients with type 2 diabetes [15] suggests that abnormal insulin-mediated suppression of plasma FFA is an early defect in those with a genetic predisposition to insulin resistance [15]. The suppressive effect of insulin on the FFA level is also reduced in nonobese insulin-resistant individuals.

Positron emission tomography (PET) scan studies using [^{18}F]-fluorodeoxyglucose with a euglycemic insulin clamp in diabetic and nondiabetic individuals have shown that there is a reduction in insulin-mediated glucose uptake in the myocardium in diabetes. Concurrent monitoring of the coronary blood flow demonstrated that this effect was not due to a reduction in perfusion, but rather to a reduction in the ability of myocardium to take up glucose under the effect of insulin.

Q: What are the glucocentric and lipocentric views of insulin resistance?

It has been suggested that there are two different defects that are responsible for impairment of glycogen synthesis, depending on the FFA concentration. Reduction in carbohydrate oxidation is responsible for only one third, while impairment of nonoxidative glucose metabolism, which mostly reflects glycogen synthesis, is responsible for two thirds of the fatty acid–dependent reduction in glucose uptake [20]. It has now been proposed that FFAs induce insulin resistance in human muscle at the level of insulin-stimulated glucose transport or phosphorylation by impairing the insulin-signaling pathway.

GLUCOCENTRIC VIEW

Previously, it was thought that FFA production from overloaded fat cells disrupted glucose homeostasis via the Randle glucose-fatty acid cycle. An elevated concentration of NEFA has been known since the 1960s to cause insulin resistance [21]. The original hypothesis, first described by Randle et al in 1963, suggested that fatty acids compete for substrate oxidation. With NEFAs acting as a competitive energy source to glucose, this can lead to defects in oxidative and nonoxidative pathways of glucose metabolism, affecting skeletal and adipose tissue. Randle et al speculated that an increase in fat oxidation may be the cause of insulin resistance in the obese.

The oxidation of FFAs was proposed to result in decreased glucose oxidation and increased intracellular citrate concentration, which would reduce glycogen and glucose uptake [17]. It was suggested that increased fatty acid oxidation would cause an increase in the mitochondrial acetyl CoA and in the reduced nicotinamide adenine dinucleotide/oxidized form of nicotinamide adenine dinucleotide ($NADH/NAD^+$) ratio, with subsequent inactivation of pyruvate dehydrogenase. In turn, this would lead to an increased intracellular citrate level. The NEFAs acting as a competitive energy source to glucose can lead to defects in oxidative and nonoxidative pathways of glucose metabolism, affecting skeletal and adipose tissue (Fig. 3.2). Reduced nicotinamide adenine dinucleotide is capable of inhibiting the citric acid cycle (urea cycle, Krebs' cycle), and the resulting accumulation of citric acid would inhibit phosphofructokinase-1 (PFK-1) and hence increase the glucose-6-phosphate. In the muscle, glucose-6-phosphate inhibits hexokinase, and the resultant rise in intracellular glucose would lead finally to decreased glucose uptake [17]. In the liver, in contrast to muscle, the increased content of glucose-6-phosphate from the reduction of glycolysis and the stimulation of gluconeogenesis should not affect glucose uptake because liver glucokinase, unlike muscle hexokinase, is not inhibited by fructose-6-phosphate. As in muscle, FFA oxidation might not be a sufficient explanation for FFA-induced changes in glucose metabolism in liver. Studies of skeletal muscle, which is responsible for the majority of whole-body insulin-mediated glucose uptake, only partially confirmed Randle's hypothesis, as FFAs reduced glucose oxidation but did not consistently reduce glucose uptake [17]. Studies show that in muscle, FFAs have effects on glucose metabolism other than or beyond that postulated by the classic Randle hypothesis (i.e., through inhibition of PFK-1 by citrate). For example, insulin-stimulated glucose uptake has been found to proceed normally for several hours after maximum inhibition of carbohydrate oxidation by fatty acids.

LIPOCENTRIC VIEW

The major factor that predisposes to the development of insulin resistance is an overabundance of circulatory fatty acids, which are derived predominantly from adipose tissue triglyceride stores released through the action of the cyclic adenosine monophosphate (cAMP)-dependent enzyme hormone–sensitive lipase and also through lipolysis of triglyceride-rich lipoproteins in tissues by the action of lipoprotein lipase. Insulin is important both for antilipolysis and for the stimulation of lipoprotein lipase. However, the most sensitive pathway of insulin action is the inhibition of lipolysis in adipose tissue. As a result, in the presence of insulin resistance, enhanced lipolysis of stored triacylglycerol molecules in adipose tissue produces more fatty acids, which further inhibit the antilipolytic effect, resulting in exaggerated lipolysis. Lipolysis is the process by which fatty acids are hydrolyzed from the intracellular triglycerides within adipose tissue that are ready for release into the circulation. The primary lipolytic agent is catecholamine. Growth hormone has a limited role, while insulin, insulin-like growth factors I and II, adenosine, prostaglandin E_1, and neuropeptide Y are all potent inhibitors. Lipogenesis is the process by which circulatory triglycerides are hydrolyzed to form NEFAs, which can be taken up by adiposities and reesterified into intracellular triglycerides. The NEFAs are transported bound to albumin. The most important pathway regulating the process of accumulating triglycerides in tissues is the lipoprotein lipase (LPL) pathway. The maintenance of triglyceride stores relies mainly on lipolysis and lipogenesis, which are important both in health and in disease.

The lipocentric hypothesis suggests that abnormalities in the fatty acid metabolism may lead to inappropriate ectopic accumulation of lipids in extraadipose tissues such as muscles, liver, and the β cells of the pancreas, which is responsible for the development of insulin resistance in corresponding sites (lipotoxicity). Lipid accumulation within monocytes and hepatocytes is strongly associated with insulin resistance in diabetics; in nondiabetic relatives of patients with type 2 diabetes, a cohort at high risk of developing diabetes; in patients with impaired glucose tolerance

[22]; and in obese children. This finding is supported by nuclear magnetic resonance (NMR) spectroscopy measurements of intramyocellular lipids (IMCLs), which correlate more closely with insulin resistance than do any other commonly measured indices, including BMI, waist/hip ratio, and total body fat [22]. In obese individuals the adipose tissue is overloaded because of excessive energy intake and decreased usage, whereas in lipodystrophy the energy intake is normal, but limited adipose tissue cannot cope with this normal intake. These individuals also tend to overeat due to low plasma leptin.

THE ROLE OF FREE FATTY ACIDS

Q: What is role of FFAs in different tissues?

Induction of Insulin Resistance by Free Fatty Acids

In a study of nondiabetic individuals, insulin resistance developed 2 to 4 hours after an acute elevation in plasma FFA level, and it took a similar amount of time to disappear after the plasma FFA level returned to normal [23]. This time gap in the development of insulin resistance after an acute rise of the plasma FFA level is suggestive of a role for some indirect mechanism. This delay is supported by the observation that acute plasma FFAs elevation increased triglyceride content in muscle cell in humans [24]. This elevation in intramyocellular triglyceride concentration occurred several hours after the elevation of FFAs and coincided with the development of insulin resistance. Boden and Laakso [24] suggest that it is probably not the accumulation of fat in muscle cells that causes insulin resistance but rather the accumulation of other metabolites, including diacylglycerol (DAG) [21], which is an intermediate of triglyceride metabolism. The routes through which FFAs can induce insulin resistance are as follows:

DAG is a potent activator of protein kinase C (PKC [the β11, αβ, and δ isoforms]. Protein kinase C is an enzyme. In the muscle, fatty acids can hinder activation of protein kinase C λ (lambda) and ζ (zeta) [25]. Also, the production of excess acyl-CoA and its derivatives such as ceramide can reduce Akt1 activation [26]. Exposing muscle cells to particular saturated FFAs inhibits insulin stimulation of Akt/protein kinase B, a serine/threonine kinase that is a central mediator of the insulin-stimulated anabolic metabolism. These saturated FFAs concomitantly induced the accumulation of ceramide and diacylglycerol, two products of fatty acyl-CoA that have been shown to accumulate in insulin-resistant tissues and to inhibit early steps in insulin signaling. Preventing de novo ceramide synthesis negated the antagonistic effect of saturated FFAs toward Akt/protein kinase B. Moreover, inducing ceramide buildup recapitulated and augmented the inhibitory effects of saturated FFAs [26]. By contrast, diacylglycerol proved dispensable for these FFA effects. This study showed that ceramide as a necessary and sufficient intermediate linking saturated fats to the inhibition of insulin signaling.

A study showed that in the liver of rats fed a high-fat diet, hepatic steatosis led to hepatic insulin resistance by stimulating gluconeogenesis and activating protein kinase C-e and c-Jun N-terminal kinase-1 (JNK1), which may interfere with tyrosine phosphorylation IRS-1 and -2 and impair the ability of insulin to activate glycogen syntheses [27].

Thus, PKC interrupts insulin signaling by serine phosphorylation of IRS-1, resulting in decreased tyrosine phosphorylation of IRS-1. In healthy individuals, a rise in the intramyocellular level of DAG paralleled an increase in PKC activity, which phosphorylates serine and threonine residues on both the insulin receptor and IRS-1. Both these molecules play a crucial role in insulin signaling. Serine phosphorylation of IRS-1 can cause its destruction and develops insulin resistance. Additionally, a change in intracellular DAG concentration is also accompanied by activation of the nuclear factor (NF)-κB pathway. Thus, activation of PKC also causes the production of inflammatory and proatherogenic proteins through activation of the inhibitor I-κBα/NF-κB pathway. Therefore, NF-κB plays an important role in the pathogenesis of coronary artery disease (CAD). Consequently, activation of NF-κB may explain the increased prevalence of vascular disease in obese individuals with type 2 diabetes. As a result, lowering the FFA level may inhibit activation of the NF-κB pathway, and this may exert beneficial effects beyond increasing insulin sensitivity and improving regulation of glucose levels [22].

There also appears to be a defect in mitochondrial oxidative phosphorylation that relates to the accumulation of triglycerides and related molecules in muscles. A study showed that in murine models of obesity, another subcellular organelle could be involved, the endoplasmic reticulum [28]. Using cell culture and mouse models, this study showed that obesity causes endoplasmic reticulum (ER) stress. This stress, in turn, leads to suppression of insulin receptor signaling through the hyperactivation of JNK and subsequent serine phosphorylation of IRS-1. Mice deficient in X-box-binding protein-1 (XBP-1), a transcription factor that modulates the ER stress response, develop insulin resistance. These findings demonstrate that ER stress is a central feature of peripheral insulin resistance and type 2 diabetes at the molecular, cellular, and organism levels.

In the liver, elevated FFAs produce increased glucose, triglycerides, VLDL cholesterol, and hyperglycemia by antagonizing the effects of insulin on endogenous glucose production. The FFAs also affect insulin secretion, but the exact nature of this relationship remains controversial.

The FFAs may induce insulin resistance by increasing oxidative stress [24]. Oxidative stress in in vitro models results in reduced responsiveness to insulin [15] and impaired insulin signaling. Additionally, the antioxidant lipoic acid prevents the induction of insulin resistance in the presence of oxidative stress [15]. It is hypothesized that activation of common stress-activated signaling pathways such as NF-κB, p38 mitogen-activated protein kinase (MAPK), and NH_2-terminal Jun kinases/stress-activated protein kinase by glucose and possibly FFAs lead to both insulin resistance and impaired insulin secretion [15]. Increased oxidative stress is the main route of action that has been suggested for the nutrient-activated pathway [15]. Increased nutrient intake enhances the production of reactive oxygen species (ROS), thus resulting in the activation of PKC isoforms, increased formation of glucose-derived advanced glycation end-products, and increased glucose flux through the aldose reductase pathway [15]. Although the relationship is well proven in the endothelial cell model of diabetic complications, the role of oxidative stress in nutrient-mediated activation of PKC will likely also prove applicable in the pathogenesis of insulin resistance [15].

Insulin Resistance and Muscle Glucose Metabolism

Skeletal muscle is responsible for the majority of insulin stimulated glucose uptake, and >80% of this glucose is stored as glycogen, which is important for whole-body glucose homeostasis. The rate of glycogen synthesis is 50% less in diabetic individuals. After skeletal muscle, the liver is the only organ that stores a significant amount of glycogen, which is also reduced in diabetics [22]. Glucose-6-phosphate is an intermediate step between glucose transport into the cell and its subsequent phosphorylation by hexokinase and glycogen synthesis. The studies show that the increase in glucose-6-phosphate concentration is slightly less in type 2 diabetics [22]. This suggests that glucose transport or phosphorylation must be the rate-limiting controlling step in insulin-stimulated glucose disposal in skeletal muscle rather than glycogen synthesis. Savage et al [22] have shown that glucose transport (as opposed to hexokinase) into the muscle is the rate-controlling step

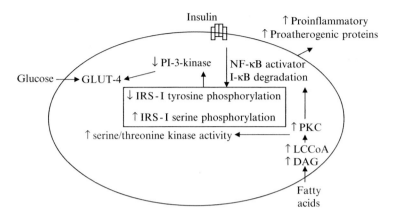

FIGURE 3.3. Mechanism of fatty acid–induced insulin resistance. Fatty acids metabolites (long-chain acyl-CoA [LCCoA]), which may accumulate within myocytes because of increased fatty acid delivery or decreased mitochondrial oxidation, activate protein kinase C (PKC), which interrupts insulin signaling by inducing serine phosphorylation of insulin receptor substrate-1 (IRS-1). This inhibits IRS-1 binding and activation of phosphatidylinositol (PI)-3-kinase, leading to reduced insulin-stimulated glucose transport. DAG, diacylglycerol. (From Boden and Laakso [24].)

for insulin-stimulated glycogen synthesis in patients with type 2 diabetes.

Fatty acid metabolites (long chain acyl-CoA [LC CoA] and DAG) accumulate within myocytes because of enhanced fatty acid availability or decreased mitochondrial oxidation. This triggers a serine/threonine kinase cascade (possible involving a novel PKC, I-κKβ, or JNK1). This subsequently induces serine/threonine phosphorylation of IRS-1 sites, thereby inhibiting IRS-1 binding and activation of PI-3-kinase, resulting in reduced insulin-stimulated glucose transport (Fig. 3.3).

MECHANISM OF LIPID ACCUMULATION IN SKELETAL MUSCLE AND LIVER

There are three ways in which lipid can accumulate in the ectopic sites: increased uptake of fatty acids, increased synthesis within corresponding tissues, and reduced fatty acid disposal by oxidation. Insulin resistance results if excess lipid accumulates in any tissue. Increased fatty acid concentration characteristically occurs in insulin-resistant individuals, the obese, type 2 diabetics, and insulin-resistant offspring of type 2 diabetics, suggesting that this may well contribute to ectopic lipid accumulation [22]. It has been hypothesized that hyperinsulinemia may have a role in promoting lipogenesis in muscle and liver by increasing sterol-regulatory element-binding protein 1c (SREBP1c) expression [29]; SREBP1c is the key transcriptional regulator of de novo lipogenesis. Lipid accumulation may be due to reduced fatty acid oxidation. Savage et al [22] showed that insulin resistance in the elderly and in lean, healthy insulin-resistant offspring of type 2 diabetics is associated with IMCL accumulation, which in turn was linked to a reduction in oxidative phosphorylation activity as assessed by magnetic resonance spectroscopy (MRS).

Liver

The main role of insulin in the liver is to control glucose production. It has been suggested that insulin suppresses glucose production by reducing the flux of amino acids and FFAs from muscle and adipose tissue to the liver, resulting in depression of gluconeogenesis. For this normal inhibitory insulin response on gluconeogenesis, insulin needs to have a normal response at the level of adipose tissue. Moreover, the ability of peripheral insulin to regulate glucose production is dependent partly on its ability to suppress FFA levels. Experiments show that hepatic insulin resistance is required for the onset of overt diabetes [30]. These studies also suggest that insulin resistance in the liver is an intrinsic abnormality in insulin signaling in the hepatocytes. Indeed, the liver might acutely affect peripheral insulin action. The mechanism by which insulin acutely (within 1 to 2 hours) suppresses hepatic glucose production is by inhibiting glycogenolysis. The FFAs produce insulin resistance in the liver by inhibiting the acute insulin suppression of glycogenolysis.

Experimental studies have shown that FFA levels per se acutely induce the expression of hepatic glucose-6-phosphatase in normal rats. Combined elevation of malonyl-CoA and cytosolic long-chain CoA may contribute to increased hepatic glucose production in obesity and type 2 diabetes. Conversely, hyperinsulinemia enhances conditions favoring FFA biosynthesis, thereby further influencing metabolic condition adversely [15]. Elevated levels of malonyl-CoA, by suppressing carnitine palmitoyl transferase-1 (CPT-1), cause a preferential flux away from FFA oxidation and in favor of esterification, with increased production of triglycerides and very low density lipopolysaccharides and aggravation of the hyperlipidemia and insulin resistance [15].

Brain

In the brain, hypothalamic resistance to central appetite-suppressing and metabolic effects of insulin may play some role in the pathogenesis of the metabolic syndrome. The insulin receptor situated in the brain is responsible for satiety associated with food. Glucose disposal in the neuron occurs in an insulin-dependent fashion. Additionally, hypothalamus and some other areas in the brain express glucose transporter GLUT-4. These areas may play an important role in hepatic glucose metabolism.

HYPERTRIGLYCERIDEMIA

Q: What is the mechanism of hypertriglyceridemia in the metabolic syndrome?

The liver becomes resistant to the inhibitory effects of insulin on VLDL secretion in the presence of hyperinsulinemia [31]. Visceral obesity and intraabdominal fat precede the development of insulin resistance, which in turn is the precursor of the following steps: (1) Visceral adipocytes become more sensitive to the metabolic effects of lipolytic hormones, glucocorticoids, and catecholamine [31]. This results in increased release of FFAs into the portal vein, which serves as a hepatic substrate for the formation of triglycerides and triglyceride-rich VLDLs. (2) There is increased production of ApoB, the major protein for LDL, and this leads to the increased synthesis and secretion of triglyceride containing VLDL-C particles [17].

In insulin resistance and type 2 diabetes, there is defective esterification and reesterification of fatty acids in adipose tissue. Possibly, there is also insulin-mediated suppression of hormone-sensitive lipase (HSL), the rate-limiting enzyme for adipose tissue triglyceride mobilization (Fig. 3.3). Enhanced lipolysis results in diversion of fat to nonadipose tissue, where it causes insulin resistance. Increased influx of NEFAs in the liver increases the size of the hepatocyte fatty acid pool. In the presence of insulin resistance, hepatic de novo lipogenesis is increased, and esterification of incoming fatty acids is relatively preferred over oxidation. Esterified fatty acids are stored as cytosolic triglycerides or diverted toward VLDL synthesis. An increased VLDL synthesis leads to increased plasma levels that release FFAs and generate remnants as a result of lipolysis by LPL. The FFAs and remnants of triglyceride-rich lipoprotein contribute to an enhanced hepatocytes fatty acid pool; thus a vicious circle sets in. The production rate of ApoB is an important regulatory step in VLDL production. Microsomal transfer protein (MTP) catalyzes the transfer of lipids to the ApoB molecule and is important factor involved in the formation of ApoB-containing lipoproteins.

De Novo Lipogenesis

The increased production of VLDL is characterized by an increased synthesis of large VLDL particles (VLDL1), rich in triglycerides and cholesterol. The VLDL1 particles are more atherogenic because they are easily taken up by the scavenger receptors of macrophages, enhancing lipid accumulation within macrophages and leading to the formation of foam cells. Glycation of apoproteins in VLDL (ApoB, ApoC, ApoE) may occur in diabetics, which may reduce VLDL binding to the apo-B,E receptors and therefore reduce catabolism. It is also suggested that glycation of ApoC-II, a cofactor of lipoprotein lipase, could contribute to lesser activation of this enzyme [32]. Chronic hyperinsulinemia and intake of carbohydrate stimulate production of newly formed fatty acids (*de novo* lipogenesis) by stimulating the activity of the lipogenic enzyme in the liver and by increasing the transcription of the genes for fatty acid synthase and acetyl-coenzyme A carboxylase [17]. This process is facilitated by increasing transcription of SREBP1c, a member of a family of regulated transcription factors [17]. Although there is downregulation of the IRS-2–mediated insulin signaling pathway in insulin-resistant states, there seems to be upregulation of SREBP1c and chronic stimulation of de novo lipogenesis in the liver, which can in turn increase the intracellular availability of triglycerides, enhancing fatty liver and resulting in VLDL formation and secretion [17]. The role of de novo synthesis is very insignificant (about 5%) in the postabsorptive state. However, it seems to be a marker of relative rate of fatty acid reesterification vs. oxidation. There is know correlation between the rate of *de novo* lipogenesis and the secretion of VLDL.

Hepatic Insulin Resistance

Insulin acutely inhibits VLDL synthesis. This effect is modified by nutritional status (fed or fasted), but this effect is lost in hyperinsulinemia associated with the metabolic syndrome, type 2 diabetes, and obesity. Peripheral tissue insulin resistance, hepatic insulin resistance/overinsulinization, or the presence of visceral obesity may have a role. The hepatic VLDL-ApoB overproduction is associated with whole-body insulin resistance and reduced hepatic insulin signaling. Lewis et al [17,33] showed that the fructose-fed hamster model was accompanied by hyperinsulinemia, increased MTP expression in the liver, and increased intracellular ApoB stability, and aided in the formation of ApoB-containing lipoprotein, leading to VLDL oversecretion. Of particular interest was the interaction of MTP abundance/activity, intracellular ApoB stability, and core lipid availability in determining the efficacy of the VLDL assembly process. Induction of insulin resistance was associated with a substantial rise in hepatic VLDL-ApoB and VLDL-triglyceride production. Increased ApoB secretion seems to be caused by enhanced intracellular stability of ApoB, an increased level of MTP, and augmented formation of VLDL particles with no apparent changes in ApoB translocation status in the endoplasmic reticulum [17]. Further studies found molecular evidence for impairment of hepatic insulin signaling and insulin resistance, including reduced tyrosine phosphorylation of the insulin recep-tors IRS-1 and -2, and suppressed activity of PI-3-kinase associated with IRS proteins [34]. It has been observed that changes in the insulin signaling pathway coincided with dramatic suppression of the ER-60 homologue. Additionally, impairment of hepatic insulin signal transduction may negate a regulatory effect of insulin on MTP expression, leading to the overexpression of this key protein, which may enable VLDL formation and secretion.

Q: What are the abnormalities of FFA metabolism in the metabolic syndrome?

The plasma FFA level is the net result of a balance between FFA release (from intravascular lipolysis of triglyceride-rich lipopro-teins and lipolysis of adipose tissue triglyceride stores) and uptake (via reesterification in adipose tissue and liver and oxidized in muscle, heart, liver, and other tissues). Different factors are impor-tant during fasting and postprandial states. During postabsorptive states the circulatory FFA level depends on the rate of FFA entry into the circulation, and during the postprandial state this depends on the rate of uptake (for reesterification, particularly adipose tissue). Postprandial FFAs may also be increased. Studies show that elevated plasma FFA is an independent predictor of progres-sion to type 2 diabetes in Caucasians and Pima Indians. The FFA level correlated with low insulin-mediated glucose disposal in first-degree relatives of type 2 diabetics [35].

Role of Hormone-Sensitive Lipase

Insulin has a potent suppressive effect on HSL, which has a crucial role in FFA release from adipose tissue. Hormone-sensitive lipase is an enzyme that is the main regulator of FFA release from adipose tissue. In insulin-resistant individuals, whether obese or not, there is a diminished suppressive effect of insulin on FFA release, which could be due to resistance of HSL to insulin. Besides, resistance to the insulin-suppressive effect on HSL is also seen postprandially in the metabolic syndrome and type 2 diabetes [17].

Adipose Tissue Uptake and Intracellular Esterification of Fatty Acids

Although insulin plays important role in the suppression of HSL, another important pathway of insulin action is in stimulating postprandial glucose uptake and FFA esterification, but Riemens et al [35] suggest that the predominant abnormality is an increased rate of release of FFA from esterification in adipose tissue. Esterification in fat cells depends on the supply of glucose-3-phosphate derived from insulin-mediated glucose uptake and glycolysis in adipose tissue. But since the insulin-mediated uptake is reduced in insulin resistance, this leads to diminished esterification. It is not clear if insulin directly stimulates the enzyme, DGAT, that is involved in the final step in triglyceride synthesis. Lipoprotein lipase plays an important role in the first step in plasma triglyceride and FFA delivery to adipocyte, especially during the postprandial state. Insulin and glucose normally stimulates adipose tissue LPL activity and reduce LPL activity in muscle. This indicates that there is preferential partitioning of lipoprotein derived from fatty acids and toward adipose tissue and away from muscle. In obesity and type 2 diabetes, insulin activation of LPL in adipose tissue is delayed, and LPL activity is delayed by hyperinsulinemia [17].

The FFAs are provided to fat cells and other tissues by chylomicrons and VLDL. They are also synthesized in the fat depots in which they are stored. They circulate in the body bound to albumin and are the major source of energy. The supply of FFAs to the tissue is regulated by lipoprotein lipase and hormone-sensitive lipase. Lipoprotein lipase is located on the surface of the endothelium of the capillaries. If hydrolyzed, the triglycerides in chylomicrons and VLDL release FFAs and glycerol, which then enter adipose tissue and are reesterified (and reassembled into new triglycerides in the fat cells). The intracellular hormone-sensitive lipase of adipose tissue catalyzes the breakdown of stored triglycerides into glycerol and fatty acids, with the latter entering the circulation.

Lipoprotein lipase plays a crucial role during the initial steps of plasma triglyceride clearance and delivery of FFAs to adipocytes, especially during the postprandial state [17]. A deficiency in CD36, a protein analogous to CD36/fatty acid transporter (FAT) in humans, has been suggested as the cause of metabolic abnormalities seen in the insulin-resistant hypertensive rats [34]. CD36 deficiency is observed in 2% to 3% of the Japanese population and may be associated with insulin resistance and dyslipidemia [17]. However, an association between CD36 deficiency and the metabolic syndrome is not yet proven.

Fat Diversion from Adipose to Nonadipose Tissue

A positive energy balance (net result of energy intake and energy expenditure) in an individual results in triglyceride accumulation in adipose tissue. This causes development of adipocyte insulin resistance and consequent diversion of fatty acids to nonadipose tissues (e.g., liver, muscle, and β cells). In addition, adipose tissue cells could adaptively limit further accumulation by becoming insulin resistant, hence diverting fat to nonadipose tissues. Cytosolic triglyceride accumulation in nonadipose tissue (e.g., liver and muscle) is linked to the development of insulin resistance in these tissues, and an attempt to protect them from energy overload. In pancreatic β cells, insulin resistance may finally cause β-cell dysfunction and damage.

It is interesting that many massively obese individuals have fewer manifestations of the metabolic syndrome, which could be explained by the theory that insulin resistance develops because of an imbalance of fat distribution between tissues [36], and that massively obese individuals probably have more efficient adipose tissue fat-storing capacity, which protects them from lipotoxicity in nonadipose tissue [17]. It seems that there is reciprocal channeling of fuels between muscle and fat when one or the other tissues become preferentially insulin resistant [17]. Downregulation of GLUT-4 and glucose transport selectively in adipose tissue have been suggested to cause insulin resistance in muscles, possibly by diverting FFAs and other fuels from adipose to nonadipose tissues [37]. However, the mechanism is not clearly understood.

Abnormal Fatty-Acid Metabolism in Skeletal Muscle

Intramyocellular triglyceride (IMTG) accumulation has been associated with muscle insulin resistance in humans [17], but the mechanism remains unclear. It is not known whether muscle triglyceride accumulation is merely a marker or if it participates in the causation of insulin resistance, because IMTG is observed in highly physically trained individuals, but it is known that muscle triglyceride may not exert adverse effects if there is a capacity for efficient lipid utilization [38]. Unlike in physically trained athletes, the muscle from obese, insulin-resistant, and type 2 diabetic individuals has a reduced capacity for uptake and oxidation of fatty acids derived from the plasma FFA pool during fasting and exercise [38]. It is possible that these changes are caused by defects of fatty acid oxidation at the CPI-1 and post–CPT-1 levels [17]. Studies suggest that impaired muscle fatty-acid oxidation is the primary defect causing the IMTG accumulation and muscle insulin resistance in individuals with type 2 diabetes and the metabolic syndrome [38]. Impaired muscle FFA oxidation in these conditions could also be due to excessive chronic exposure to FFAs because the elevation of malonyl-CoA due to energy excess has been associated with reduced muscle fat oxidation through inhibition of CPI-1 [39]. Improvement in insulin resistance with reduction of obesity is associated with a reduction of lipid oxidation relative to carbohydrate oxidation [40].

Skeletal muscle has a high fractional extraction of FFAs in the postabsorptive state, and lipid oxidation is responsible for the major source of energy [38]. It has been suggested that muscle fatty acid binding and transport proteins (FABPs) are altered in obesity and type 2 diabetes but not in the glucose-tolerant obese person [41]. Studies show that excessive FFA delivery to muscle from the circulation could be the cause of muscle triglyceride accumulation [42]. Also any extramuscular defect of fatty acid metabolism could lead to intramyocellular triglyceride accumulation and the skeletal muscle lipotoxic effects seen in obesity and type 2 diabetes [43].

Q: How does atherogenesis occur in the metabolic syndrome when low-density lipoprotein cholesterol is normal?
Although LDL cholesterol may be normal in some patients with the metabolic syndrome, there are other multiple atherogenic alterations that predispose to CVD. Three explanations support this finding: First, the levels of VLDL particles are raised, and the particles can enter the vessel wall and accumulate in atherosclerotic plaques. Also, VLDL, by virtue of receiving CETP-transferred cholesteryl esters, is able to deliver more cholesterol per particle to the vessel wall [44]. Furthermore, increased VLDL secretion can lead to postprandial hyperlipidemia by providing competition for the chylomicron clearance pathways. Postprandial hyperlipidemia is independently associated with CVD. Second, low HDL cholesterol and ApoA-1 levels result in fewer HDL particles that are participating in cholesterol efflux from peripheral tissues, which is the initial step in reverse cholesterol transport. High-density lipoprotein cholesterol, by virtue of having fewer HDL particles, is unable to exert direct antiatherogenic actions at the vessel wall, including its antioxidant properties. Scavenger receptor B1 (SRB1), seems to mediate the selective delivery of HDL cholesteryl esters to the liver (delivery of core lipid by the HDL particle without endocystosis and degradation of the whole particle), thus targeting that cholesterol for excretion via the biliary pathway [44]. The CETP-mediated transfer of HDL cholesterol esters to VLDL enables enrichment of an atherogenic lipoprotein with cholesterol and also diverts that cholesterol from the specific reverse

cholesterol transport pathway. Hypertriglyceridemia leading to low HDL cholesterol and increased small, dense LDL particles is due mainly to the actions of CEPT. Third, small, dense LDL particles are known to be more atherogenic than an equal number of larger more cholesteryl ester-rich LDL, due to their susceptibility to oxidation and their ability to penetrate and adhere to the arterial wall.

POSTPRANDIAL GLYCEMIA

Q: What is the importance of postprandial glycemia clinically?
Strong circumstantial evidence links raised postprandial glycemia (PPG) with insulin resistance, vascular endothelial dysfunction, and CVD. It is also possible that PPG might accelerate β-cell decline (and atherosclerosis) via exposure to a prolonged stressful tide of glucose and lipids after eating. During the progression from normal glucose tolerance to overt diabetes, PPG levels rise, preceded by the fasting glucose rise. In type 2 diabetes, the postprandial rise in glucose is higher and more sustained compared with individuals without diabetes. The PPG is observed to contribute to insulin resistance and reduced secretion of insulin [45]. For instance, if PPG remains high for more than 2 hours, postprandial insulin receptors are downregulated, contributing to increased insulin resistance [37]. Due to increased islet glucose concentration, there is a decrease of insulin release, with prolonged hyperglycemia and accelerated loss of β-cell function (glucotoxicity). High levels of FFAs, which occur in obesity, further contribute to raised PPG by impairing β-cell function (lipotoxicity) and can induce β-cell apoptosis [46]. It has been suggested that intestinal FABPs could contribute to postprandial lipid abnormalities, insulin resistance, and diabetes [47].

Postprandial Glycemia Contribution to Hemoglobin A_{1c}

Hemoglobin A_{1c} (HbA_{1c}) represents an integration of both fasting and postprandial glycemia [48]. However, in early stages small increases in HbA_{1c} are associated with increased PPG, while the fasting level remains normal. Post-lunch glucose levels have a strong relationship to HbA_{1c}, and fasting plasma glucose alone underestimates HbA_{1c}. Postprandial hyperglycemia itself is an independent risk factor for CVD. The Diabetes Epidemiology Collaborative Analysis of Diagnostic Criteria in Europe (DECODE) study showed that the 2-hour postglucose challenge level was associated with mortality even in those with a normal fasting glucose [49]. Some studies show that the 2-hour post-glucose level is a direct predictor of CVD, independent of other risk factors [50]. However, some authors believe that the PPG is instead a marker for insulin resistance. Many CVD risk factors are altered in the postprandial phase, with changes including the glycation of lipoproteins, the generation of free radicals, increased oxidative stress, increased coagulability, high levels of circulating adhesion molecules and inflammatory cytokines, and decreased nitric oxide (NO) production [51]. Macrovascular complication can be seen in impaired glucose tolerance (IGT). A raised PPG is also a marker of reduced β-cell function, which is associated with proinsulin, which in turn plays a role in the development of CVD.

Overall, there is good evidence to support the idea that targeting PPG excursion is clinically beneficial. For example, in a comparison between treatments with a prandial glucose regulator or a sulfonylureas over 12 months, there was greater regression in carotid intimal media thickness (IMT) in the prandial glucose regulator group along with lower PPG [52]. Lowering of the HbA_{1c} level reduces microvascular and macrovascular complications. A therapeutic intervention aimed at reducing the PPG has been shown to be more effective in reducing HbA_{1c} than other treatments. For example, type 2 diabetic patients inadequately controlled on sulfonylureas were randomized to receive glyburide in combination with insulin lispro 1 (to target PPG), metformin (to target pre-meal blood glucose levels), or neutral protamine Hagedorn (NPH) insulin at night (to target fasting blood glucose). All therapies improve HbA_{1c} but glyburide plus insulin lispro was most effective [53].

GROWTH HORMONES

Q: What is the role of growth hormones in the pathway of the metabolic syndrome?
There are many similarities between Cushing syndrome and the metabolic syndrome. It has been suggested that some components of cortisol production or signaling may be involved in the pathogenesis of the metabolic syndrome [6]. A combination of factors may be involved, but the exact mechanism is not known. Some of the actions of glucocorticoids on carbohydrate and lipid metabolism are antagonist to that of insulin principally. Glucocorticoid hormones increase the sensitivity of adipocytes to adrenaline, to increase lipolysis, and to skeletal muscle, to release lactate. Glucocorticoids acutely activate lipolysis in adipose tissue. It is hypothesized that a neuroendocrine disturbance involving the hypothalamic-pathway axis (HPA) may be involved [54]. Altered cellular glucocorticoid

hormone action may be responsible for some features of the metabolic syndrome. Genetic polymorphisms of the glucocorticoid receptor (GR) alter glucocorticoid hormone action and are associated with the metabolic syndrome [55]. However, the relative contribution of the GR genotype to blood pressure appears to be small. Subsequently it is suggested that tissue-specific molecular determinants of glucocorticoid hormone action may be the underlying cause of a modest alteration in glucocorticoid hormone action in the pathogenesis of metabolic syndrome [56].

In muscle cell culture, Byrne and Wild [6] have shown that GR messenger RNA (mRNA) levels are positively correlated with the degree of insulin resistance. These data suggest a strong link between tissue sensitivity to glucocorticoid hormone and both resistance to insulin-mediated glucose uptake in skeletal muscle and obesity. 11β-hydroxysteroid dehydrogenase (11β-HSD) has been mentioned to play some role [57]. There are two distinct isoforms of 11β-HSD, namely type 1 (11β-HSD-1), which encodes relatively low-affinity NADP/NADPH-dependent 11-dehydrogenase and oxo-reductase activity, and type 2 (11β-HSD-2), which encodes high affinity NAD-dependent 11-dehydrogenase activity. Their different kinetic characteristics suggest distinct physiological roles [6]. Fetal overexposure to increased concentrations of glucocorticoids may affect the subsequent development of the metabolic syndrome [58]. Glucocorticoids slow fetal growth and may alter the size of the placenta, depending on the dose and the timing of exposure. A rise in systolic blood pressure in the adult offspring has been observed months after this exposure to glucocorticoid therapy.

References

1. Hales C, Barker D. Type 2 diabetes mellitus: the thrifty phenotype hypothesis. Diabetologia 1992;35:595–601.
2. Laakso M. Gene variants, insulin resistance, and dyslipidemia. Curr Opin Lipidol 2004;2:115–120.
3. Savage DB, Tam GD, Acerini CL, et al. Human metabolic syndrome resulting from dominant-negative mutations in the nuclear receptor PPARγ. Diabetes 2003;52:910–917.
4. Farooq IS, O'Rahilly S, Monogenic obesity in humans. Annu Rev Med 2005;56:443–458.
5. Gibson WT, Farooqi IS, Moreau M, et al. J Clin Endocrinol Metab 2004;89:4821–4826.
6. Byrne CD, Wild SH. The Metabolism Syndrome. New York: John Wiley & Sons, 2005.
7. Kissebah AH, Sonnenberg G, Myklebust J, et al. Quantitative trait loci on chromosome 3 and 17 influence phenotypes of the metabolic syndrome. Proc Natl Acad Sci USA 2000;97:14478–14483.

8. Sarkkinen E, Korhonen M, Krkkila A, et al. Effects of apo E polymorphism on serum lipid response to the separate modification of dietary fat and dietary cholesterol. Am J Clin Nutr 1998;68:1215–1222.

9. Wilson PW, Schaefer ES, Larson MG, et al. Apo E alleles and risk of coronary disease. Atheroscler Thromb Vasc Biol 1996;16:1250–1255.

10. Song Y, Niu T, Manson JE, et al. Are variants in the Calpain10 gene related to risk of type 2 diabetes? Am J Hum Genet 2004;74:208–222.

11. Weedon MN, Frayling TM, Shields B, et al. Genetic regulation of birth weight and fasting glucose by a common polymorphism in the islet cell promoter of the glucokinase gene. Diabetes 2005;54:576–581.

12. Laakso M. Gene variants, insulin resistance, and dyslipidemia. Curr Opin Lipidol 2004;2:115–120.

13. Florez JC. Phenotypic consequences of the PPARγ Pro12A1a polymorphism. J Clin Endocrinol Metab 2004;89:4234–4237.

14. Eckel RH, Grundy SM, Zimmet P. The metabolic syndrome. Lancet 2005;365:9468–9415.

15. Khan CR, Weir GC, King GL. Joslin's Diabetes Mellitus. Philadelphia: Lippincott Williams & Wilkins, 2005.

16. Randle PJ, Garland PB, Hales CN, et al. The glucose fatty acid cycle. Lancet 1963;1:785–789.

17. Lewis GF, Carpentier A, Adeli K, et al. Disordered fat storage and mobilization in the pathogenesis of insulin resistance and type 2 diabetes. Endocr Rev 2002;23:201–229.

18. Grundy SM. Does the metabolic syndrome exist? Diabetes Care 2006;29:1689–1692.

19. Grundy SM, Brewer HB, Cleeman JI, et al. Definition of metabolic syndrome. Circulation 2004;109:433–438.

20. Kahn BB, Flier JS. Obesity and insulin resistance. J Clin Invest 2000;106:473–481.

21. Boden G. Role of fatty acids in the pathogenesis of insulin resistance and NIDDM. Diabetes 1966;45:3–10.

22. Savage DB, Petersen KF, Shulman GI. Mechanisms of insulin resistance in humans and possible links with inflammation. Hypertension 2005;45:828–837.

23. Homko CJ, Cheug P, Boden G, et al. Effects of FFAs on glucose uptake and utilization in healthy women. Diabetes 2003;52:487–491.

24. Boden G, Laakso M. Lipid and glucose in type 2 diabetes. Diabetes Care 2004;27:2253–2259.

25. Kim YB, Shulman, Kahn BB. Fatty acid infusion selectively impairs insulin action on Akt1 and protein kinase C lambda/zeta but not on glycogen synthase kinase-3. J Biol Chem 2002;277:32915–32922.

26. Chaves JA, Knotts TA, Wang LP, et al. A role for ceramide, but not diacylglycerol, in the antagonism of insulin signal transduction by saturated fatty acids. J Biol Chem 2003;278:10297–10303.

27. Samuel VT, Liu ZX, Qu X, et al. Mechanism of hepatic insulin resistance in non-alcoholic fatty liver disease. J Biol Chem 2004;279:32345–32353.

28. Ozcan U, Cao Q, Yilmaz E, et al. Endoplasmic reticulum stress links obesity, insulin action and type 2 diabetes. Science 2004;306: 457–461.

29. Shimomura I, Matsuda M, Hammer RE, et al. Decreased IRS-2 and increased SREBO-1c lead to mixed insulin resistance and sensitivity in livers of lipodystrophic and ob/ob mice. Mol Cell 2000;6:77–86.

30. Lauro D, Kido Y, Castle AL, et al. Impaired glucose intolerance in mice with a targeted impairment of insulin action in muscle and adipose tissue. Nat Genet 1998;20:294–298.

31. Kolovou GD, Anagnostopoulou KK, Cokkinos DV. Pathophysiology of dyslipidemia in the metabolic syndrome. Postgrad Med J 2005;81: 358–366.

32. Saheki S, Hitsumoto Y, Murase M, et al. In vitro degradation of VLDL from diabetic patient by lipoprotein lipase. Clin Chim Acta 1993;217: 105–114.

33. Taghibiglou C, Carpenter A, Vanlderstine SC, Lewis GF, et al. Mechanism of hepatic VLDL overproduction in insulin resistance. J Biol Chem 2000;275:8416–8425.

34. Taghibiglou C, Van Inderstine S, Chen B, et al. Hepatic VLDL overproduction and reduced apo B degradation in an animal model of insulin resistance, the fructose-fed hamster, is associated with suppression of intracellular levels of ER-60 protease. Circulation 2000;102:11–88.

35. Riemens SC, Sluiter WJ, Dullaart RP. Enhanced escape of NEFAs from tissue uptake. Diabetologia 2000;43:416–426.

36. Shulman GI. Cellular mechanism of insulin resistance. J Clin Invest 2000;106:171–176.

37. Abdel ED, Peroni O, Kim JK, et al. Adipose-selecting targeting of the GLUT 4 gene impairs insulin action in muscle and liver. Nature 2000;409:729–733.

38. Kelley DE, Goodpaster BH. Skeletal muscle triglyceride. An aspect of regional adiposity and insulin resistance. Diabetes Care 2001;24:933–941.

39. Baveholm PN, Pigon J, Saha AK, et al. Fatty acid oxidation and the regulation of malonyl-CoA in human muscle. Diabetes 2000;49: 1078–1083.

40. Beneditte G, Mingrone G, Marcoccia S, et al. Body composition and energy expenditure after weight loss following bariatric surgery. J Am Coll Nutr 2000;19:270–274.

41. Simoneau JA, Veerkamp JH, Turcotte LP, et al. Markers of capacity to utilize fatty acids in human skeletal muscle: relation to insulin resistance and obesity and effects of weight loss. FASEB J 1999;13: 2051–2060.

42. Boden G, Lebed B, Schatz M, et al. Effects of acute changes of plasma free fatty acids on intramyocellular fat content and insulin resistance in healthy subjects. Diabetes 2001;50:1612–1617.

43. Sparks JD, Sparks CE. Insulin regulation of triacylgycerol-rich lipoprotein synthesis and secretion. Biochim Biophys Acta 1994;1215: 9–32.

44. Acton S. Indentification of scavenger receptor SR-B1 as a high density lipoprotein receptor. Science 1996;27:460–461.

45. Bell DS. Importance of postprandial glucose control. South Med J 2001;94(8):804–809.

46. Robertson RP, Harmon J, Tran PO, et al. Beta-cell glucose toxicity, lipotoxicity, and chronic oxidative stress in type 2 diabetes. Diabetes 2004;53(suppl 1):S119–124.

47. Hagele RA. A review of intestinal fatty acid binding protein gene variation and the plasma lipoprotein response to dietary components. Clin Biochem 1998;31:609–612.

48. Ward H. Importance of managing postprandial glycemia in type 2 diabetes. Diabetes Dig 2006;5(3, suppl):3–5.

49. DECODE Study Group. Comparison of WHO and ADA diagnostic criteria. Lancet 1999;354(9179):G17–21.

50. Meigs JB, Nathan DM, D'Agustino RB Sr, et al. The Framingham Offspring Study. Diabetes Care 2002;25(10):1845–1850.

51. Ceriello A. Postprandial hypoglycemia and diabetes complications. Diabetes 2005;54(1):1–7.

52. Esposito K, Glugliano D, Nappo F, et al. Regression of carotid atherosclerosis by control of postprandial hyperglycemia in type 2 diabetes mellitus. Circulation 2004;110(2):214–219.

53. Bastyr EJ 3rd, Stuart CA, Brodows RG, et al. Therapy focused on lowering postprandial glucose, not fasting glucose, may be superior for lowering HbA1c. Diabetes Care 2000;23(9):1236–1241.

54. Bjorntorp P. Insulin resistance: the consequences of a neuroendocrine disturbance. Int J Obes Relat Metab Disord 1995;19(suppl 1):S6–S10.

55. Weaver JU, Hitman GA, Kopelman, et al. An association between a Bell restriction fragment length polymorphism of the glucocorticoid receptor locus and hyperinsulinaemia in obese women. J Mol Endocrinal 1992;9(3):295–300.

56. Pariarelli M, Holloway CD, Fraser R, et al. Glucocorticoid receptor polymorphism, skin vasoconstriction, and other metabolic intermediate phenotypes in normal human subjects. J Clin Endocrinal Metab 1998;83:1846–1852.

57. Seckel JR, Walker BR. 11B-Hydroxysteroid dehydrogenase type 1 as a modular of glucocorticoid action: from metabolism memory. Trends Endocrinol Metab 2004;15(9):418–424.

58. Langley-Evans SC. Intrauterine programming of hypertension by glucocorticoids. Life Sci 1997;60(15):1213–1221.

Chapter 4
Clinical Diagnosis of the Metabolic Syndrome

Q: What are the similarities and differences in the clinical diagnostic criteria of the World Health Organization and the Adult Treatment Panel-III?

In 2001, the National Cholesterol Education Program's (NCEP) Adult Treatment Panel (ATP-III) [1] published their criteria for the diagnosis of the metabolic syndrome, based on the measurements (Table 4.1) of three or more of the following: waist circumference, fasting glucose, blood pressure, triglycerides, and low HDL-C. The goal of the ATP-III was focused less on type 2 diabetes and more on cardiovascular disease (CVD) risk and primary prevention in individuals with multiple risk factors. Therefore, the ATP-III viewed the metabolic syndrome as representing "multiple, interrelated factors that raised CVD risk," and the incriminating causes were overweight/obesity, physical inactivity, and genetic factors. The features that were considered relevant in this context are abdominal obesity, atherogenic dyslipidemia, hypertension, glucose intolerance, and prothrombotic and proinflammatory states. The clinical criteria reflect also the ATP-III viewpoint that the syndrome increased CVD risk at any given low-density lipoprotein (LDL) cholesterol level, and that it should be a secondary target of therapy in cholesterol management. In doing so, the ATP-III intend to identify people at higher long-term risk for CVD who warranted clinical lifestyle intervention to reduce the risk. The ATP-III criteria included no single factor for diagnosis but rather required the presence of three of five factors (Table 4.1).

Although the ATP-III did not make any particular risk factor a prerequisite for the diagnosis of the metabolic syndrome, it prioritized abdominal obesity as a very important underlying risk factor, as it is mentioned first in the diagnostic criteria. Its cutoff points for abdominal obesity were derived from the definition of the 1998 National Institute of Health Obesity Clinical Guidelines: waist circumference (WC) of ≥102 cm (≥40 inches) for men and ≥88 cm

TABLE 4.1. Adult Treatment Panel (ATP-III) 2004 diagnostic criteria of metabolic syndrome

Risk factor	Cutoff point
Waist circumference	>102 cm (>40 inches) in men, >88 cm (>35 inches) in women
Triglycerides	≥150 mg/dL (1.7 mmol/L)
Low HDL cholesterol	
Men	<40 mg/dL (1.03 mmol/L) in men,
Women	<50 mg/dL (1.3 mmol/L)
Blood pressure	≥130/85 mm Hg or on antihypertensive drug
Fasting glucose	≥100 mg/dL (5.6 mmol/L), includes diabetes

Source: Grundy et al. [2]

(≥35 inches) for women. However, these measurements were not made prerequisite because lesser degrees of abdominal girth are often associated among South Indians. Besides, these cut points also identify approximateiy the upper quartile of the United States population. Interestingly, insulin resistance is not a prerequisite, though most individuals have it. The cutoff points for several characteristics are less stringent, indicating that the ATP-III considers that even marginal multiple risk factors can confer a significant increase risk of CVD.

The mere presence of type 2 diabetes does not confirm the diagnosis of clinical syndrome. In addition to raised blood glucose, two other characteristics need to be present. The ATP-III noted that direct measurement of insulin resistance was painstaking and not well standardized. The ATP-III, like the World Health Organization (WHO), but unlike the European Group for the Study of Insulin Resistance (EGIR) and the American Association of Clinical Endocrinologist (AACE), approved a diagnosis of the metabolic syndrome in the presence of type 2 diabetes because of the high risk for CVD among multiple risk factor patients with diabetes [2]. Some individuals manifest symptoms of insulin resistance with only moderately increased WC (i.e., 94 to 101 cm in men or 80 to 87 cm in women).

Grundy et al [2] suggest that the characteristic that predisposes to insulin resistance and metabolic abnormality in such subjects are (1) a family history of type 2 diabetes in first-degree relatives before the age of 60 years, (2) polycystic ovary syndrome (PCOS), (3) fatty liver disease, (4) C-reactive protein (CRP) ≥3 mg/L (if measured), (5) microalbuminuria (if detected), (6) impaired glucose tolerance (IGT) (if measured), and (7) elevated total apolipoprotein B (ApoB) (if measured). Grundy et al further advise that if the patients who have only moderately increased WC meet two other criteria of the ATP-III, then consideration should be given to managing them similarly with three ATP-III risk factors.

WORLD HEALTH ORGANIZATION CRITERIA

In 1999, the WHO proposed the diagnostic criteria required for the diagnosis of type 2 diabetes and the metabolic syndrome. While the ATP-III listed abdominal obesity as its priority, the WHO has given importance to insulin resistance, and it is a prerequisite for the diagnosis, emphasizing that insulin resistance is the primary cause of this syndrome. This classification was intended for individuals who are likely candidates for diabetes, as manifested by IGT, impaired fasting glucose (IFG), or insulin resistance (measured by the hyperinsulinemic euglycemic clamp). The WHO stated that each component conveyed greater CVD risk, but when combined, the components become more powerful. Therefore, the aim for diagnosing the metabolic syndrome was to identify patients at higher CVD risk. There are some significant differences from the diagnostic criteria of the ATP-III (Table 4.2):

TABLE 4.2. World Health Organization criteria of diagnosis for metabolic syndrome

Risk factor	Cutoff point
Insulin resistance	IGT, IFG, type 2 diabetes, or those with NFG (<110 mg/dL), glucose uptake below the lowest quartile for background population under investigation under hyperinsulinemic euglycemic conditions *Plus any 2 of the following:*
Blood pressure	≥140 mm Hg systolic or ≥90 mm Hg diastolic or on antihypertensive
Plasma triglyceride	≥150 mg/dL (≥1.7 mmol/L)
Plasma HDL-C	<35 mg/dL (<0.9 mmol/L) in men or <39 mg/dL (1.0 mmol/L) in women
Obesity	BMI >30 and/or waist/hip ratio >0.9 in men, >0.85 in women
Microalbuminuria	Urinary albumin excretion rate ≥20 μg/min or albumin/creatine ratio ≥30 mg/g

IGF, impaired glucose tolerance; IFG, impaired fasting glucose; NFG, normal fasting glucose.
Source: Alberti and Zimmet [4].

- The diagnostic criteria include higher blood pressure.
- Obesity is measured by body mass index (BMI) or waist/hip ratio vs. the ATP-III measures of WC.
- In those with normal fasting blood glucose, routine glucose tolerance is required.
- The diagnostic criteria include urinary albumin excretion and albumin creatinine ratio (indicating microalbuminuria).
- Insulin resistance can be recognized by the criteria listed in Table 4.2.
- IGT is included here but not in the ATP-III.

The WHO criteria allow the diagnosis of the metabolic syndrome to be applied to individuals with type 2 diabetes who otherwise met the requirements of this syndrome. The WHO thought that type 2 diabetics often have a clustering of CVD risk factors, which puts them at a particularly high risk for CVD.

Q: What are the similarities and differences in the various versions of the diagnostic criteria?
Only the WHO and the AACE diagnostic criteria included the oral glucose tolerance test (OGTT) or the 2-hour post–75-g glucose challenge, which naturally has its pros and cons. The ATP-III did not include either of these tests as they entail added inconvenience and cost in clinical practice. Besides, their added value for CVD risk prediction appears to be small. However, clinicians should exercise their discretion in diagnosing individuals without diabetes but with two or more metabolic risk factors. The advantages of performing an oral glucose tolerance (OGTT) include the following: (1) The test enables the detection of another metabolic factor in an individual without IFG but whose OGTT revealed IGT. (2) The IGT, when added to the ATP-III criteria, increases the prevalence of the metabolic syndrome among individuals over 50 years of age by 5%. (3) The presence of postprandial hyperglycemia in patients with IFG indicates a high-risk condition for CVD.

INTERNATIONAL DIABETES FEDERATION CRITERIA
In 2005, the International Diabetes Federation (IDF) published their diagnostic version. This was the result of a consensus conference organized by the IDF in which 21 participants from Europe, North and South America, Asia, Australia, and Africa were invited. This group included several members of the original WHO consulting group. There were only minor differences among the versions of the IDF, the ATP-III, and the WHO, and they share

one major feature: neither the individual components selected to serve as criteria nor the specific cutoff points are the result of prospective studies [3]. However, the criteria reflected the collective viewpoint of the participants.

The IDF agreed with the ATP-III that the ATP-III definition of the metabolic syndrome was simple and correctly considered that abdominal obesity was highly correlated with insulin resistance; so the laborious measurement of insulin was considered unnecessary. Consequently, the IDF considered obesity as a prerequisite and the presence of two other factors from the ATP-III criteria sufficient for the diagnosis (Table 4.3). However, the IDF emphasized ethnic differences in the correlation between abdominal obesity and other metabolic risk factors. In the IDF version, even if an individual manifests all of these abnormalities and also has type 2 diabetes, he or she would not be deemed to have the metabolic syndrome if the WC does not exceed the requirement.

There are two basic differences among the IDF, ATP-III, and WHO versions. One major difference is the way they are organized. The ATP-III criteria do not distinguish qualitatively among

TABLE 4.3. Diagnostic criteria of the International Diabetic Federation

Central obesity: WC ethnicity-specific values	Europid* men ≥94 cm, women ≥80 cm; South Asians** men ≥90 cm, women ≥80 cm Japanese men ≥85 cm, women ≥90 cm
Plus any two of the following:	
High triglycerides	≥150m mg/dL (1.7 mmol/L) or on medication for lipid disorder
Low HDL-C	<40 mg/dL (1.03 mmol/L) in men/ <50 mg/dL (1.3 mmol/L in women or on medication for this lipid abnormality
High blood pressure	Systolic ≥130 mm Hg or diastolic ≥85 mm Hg or on medication for blood pressure
High impaired fasting glucose	≥100 mg/dL (5.6 mmol/L) or previously diagnosed type 2 diabetes

WC, waist circumference
*Applies to Saharan African, East Mediterranean, and Middle East (Arab) population.
**Applies to Chinese, South and Central American population.
Source: Zimmet P, Alberti G, Shaw J. A new IDF worldwide definition of the metabolic syndrome: the rational and the results. Diabetes Voice 2005;50(3):31.

its components, as the combination of three of five criteria conveys that each component has the same adverse effects, which is supported by a recent statement by the American Heart Association (AHA) and the National Heart, Lung, and Blood Institute (NHLBI) that there is no common cause of the metabolic syndrome [3]. The WHO requires evidence of insulin resistance, but the IDF's fundamental criterion is an ethnicity-adjusted degree of abdominal obesity.

The other major difference among the three versions is related to excess obesity. The WHO and the AACE view the BMI as only an ancillary criterion, and the requirement can be fulfilled by either a certain degree of overall obesity, as measured by the BMI, or an excess waist/hip ratio, which is an index of abdominal obesity. In contrast, there is a greater emphasis on central obesity (as measured by waist circumference) in the ATP-III, IDF, and EGIR criteria. The IDF defines WC according to ethnicity, and the ATP-III has also included this concept indirectly by stating that for some insulin resistance–prone individuals, the lower cutoff points can be used. With recent modifications in the diagnostic criteria, the ATP-III has come fairly close to the IDF requirements; therefore, it is anticipated that for the most part an individual will be diagnosed by either definition [2].

The clinical criteria of the ATP-III, the WHO, and the IDF include diabetes, whereas the criteria of the AACE and the EGIR do not. Furthermore, IGT is included by the WHO, the EGIR, and the AACE, but not by the IDF and the ATP-III. Interestingly, microalbuminuria is required only by the WHO definition.

AMERICAN HEART ASSOCIATION AND NATIONAL HEART, LUNG, AND BLOOD INSTITUTE STATEMENT

At present, the AHA/NHLBI, unlike the IDF, support the ATP-III criteria except for minor modifications (Table 4.4). The AHA/NHLBI agreed that the ATP-III criteria are simple to use in the clinical setting and have the advantage of avoiding depending on a single cause. The AHA/NHLBI reduced the threshold for IGF from 110 to 100 mg/dL, based on the present evidence of the America Diabetic Association (ADA).

AMERICAN ASSOCIATION OF CLINICAL ENDOCRINOLOGIST CRITERIA

In 2003, the AACE modified the ATP-III criteria and emphasized insulin resistance as the primary metabolic risk factor. Like the EGIR, the AACE use the term *insulin resistance syndrome*. The criteria put forward by the AACE are a hybrid of the WHO and the

TABLE 4.4. American Heart Association/National Heart, Lung, and Blood Institute diagnostic criteria of metabolic syndrome: any three of the five criteria

Risk factor	Cutoff point
Waist circumference* (WC)	≥102 cm (≥40 in) men, ≥88 cm (≥35 in) in women, lower cutoff points for insulin-resistant person or ethnic groups (based on clinical judgment)
Triglycerides (TG)#	≥150 mg/dL(1.7 mmol/L) or on drug therapy for raised TG
Low HDL-cholesterol	<40 mg/dL (1.03 mmol/L) in men
	<50 mg/dL (1.3 mmol/L) in women or on HDL-C lowering therapy#
Blood pressure	≥130 mm Hg systolic or ≥85 mm Hg diastolic blood pressure or on antihypertensive drug therapy
Fasting glucose	≥100 mg/dL (5.6 mmol/L) or on drug therapy for raised blood glucose

*Some U.S. adults of non-Asian origin (white, black, Hispanic) with marginally increased WC (e.g., 94–101 cm [37–39 in] in men and 80–87 cm [30–34 in] in women) may have strong genetic contribution to insulin resistance and should benefit from changes in lifestyle habits, similar to men with categorical increases in WC. Lower WC cutoff points (i.e., ≥90 cm [35 in] in men and ≥80 cm [31 in] in women) appear to be appropriate for Asian Americans.
#Fibrates and nicotinic acid are most commonly used drugs for elevated triglyceride and low HDL.
Source: Courtesy of Dr. Daniel Levy, NHLBI.

ATP-III criteria [4]. In fact, there is no defined number of risk factors specified, and the diagnosis depends on the clinical judgment of the clinician. Major criteria are IGT, elevated triglycerides, low HDL cholesterol, elevated blood pressure, and obesity (Table 4.5), but no specific criteria are required for the diagnosis. The AACE advised that other factors should be taken into account by clinicians, including a family history of CVD or type 2 diabetes, PCOS, and hyperuricemia. By the AACE definition, once a person develops type 2 diabetes, the term *insulin resistance* no longer applies. Like the WHO criteria, the AACE advised performing a GTT if an abnormality is clinically suspected, even though the fasting glucose is normal. The IDF, AACE, and EGIR use the term *insulin resistance syndrome*.

TABLE 4.5. American Association of Clinical Endocrinology diagnostic criteria of insulin resistance syndrome

Risk factor	Cutoff point
Overweight/obesity	BMI ≥25
Elevated triglycerides	≥150 mg/dL (1.7 mmol/L)
Low HDL	men <40 mg/dL (1.03 mmol/L)
	women <50 mg/dL (1.3 mmol/L)
Elevated blood pressure	≥130/85 mm Hg
2-hour post–glucose challenge	>140 mg/dL (7.8 mmol/L)
Fasting glucose	110–126 mg/dL (6.1–7.0 mmol/L) but not diabetes
Other risk factors*	Family history of type 2 diabetes, hypertension or CVD; PCOS, sedentary lifestyle, advancing age, high risk ethnic group, acanthosis nigricans

CVD, cardiovascular disease; PCOS, polycystic ovary syndrome.

EUROPEAN GROUP FOR STUDY OF INSULIN RESISTANCE CRITERIA

In 1999, EGIR proposed modifications to the WHO definition but still preferred to use the term *insulin resistance syndrome* rather than *metabolic syndrome*. The EGIR also believed that insulin resistance is the major cause of this syndrome and therefore required evidence of it in their criteria for diagnosis. According to their criteria, plasma insulin levels in the upper quartile of the population defined insulin resistance. The EGIR placed more emphasis on abdominal obesity than did the WHO, and also excluded type 2 diabetes as one of the criteria required for diagnosis, reasoning that insulin resistance is primarily a risk for type 2 diabetes (Table 4.6).

Q: Does the metabolic syndrome have a common pathological cause?

The criteria required by the three major versions (ATP-III, WHO, IDF) for the diagnosis of the metabolic syndrome are very similar. The fact that the ATP-III has given equal importance to its five criteria indicates the panel's view that the cluster of abnormalities probably has more than one cause [3]. Apparently, how-soever similar the components of various diagnostic versions may appear, it cannot be denied that the related abnormalities that make up all three versions of the metabolic syndrome criteria have more than one cause. For instance, there is more than one

TABLE 4.6. European Group for the Study of Insulin Resistance criteria for the diagnosis of metabolic syndrome (1999)

Insulin resistance	Presence of fasting hyperinsulinemia (i.e., among the highest 25% of nondiabetic population
Plus any two of the following:	
Central obesity	Waist circumference ≥94 cm (men), ≥80 cm (women)
Dyslipidemia	Triglycerides ≥150 mg/dL (≥1.0 mmol/L) and/or HDL-C <39 mg/dL (<1.0 mmol/L)
Hypertension	Blood pressure ≥140/90 mm Hg or on antihypertensive
Fasting glucose	IFG (≥110 mg/dL) (≥6.1 mmol/L) or IGT (but not diabetes)

To convert serum triglycerides from mg/dL to mmol/L multiply by 0.0113. To convert HDL-C from mg/dL to mmol/L multiply by 0.0259.

cause that is implicated in hypertension. This question then arises: If any component of the metabolic syndrome has underlying multiple causes, does that mean that there could not be a common physiological event that greatly increases the possibility that a person will undergo the changes that can lead to a diagnosis of the metabolic syndrome? Gerald Reaven [3] proposes that the answer is no. He further reasons that the clustering of abnormalities that constitute components of the three major versions could not evolve accidentally, and that insulin resistance as a consequence of defective insulin action plays a fundamental role in the development of CVD via factors that make up all versions of the metabolic syndrome criteria.

The failure of international medical associations to agree on the criteria required for the diagnosis of the metabolic syndrome has raised some questions about the validity of this terminology. In the forefront, Reaven [3] has argued against this definition of the metabolic syndrome with reasoning that he has eloquently put forward in a recent article. He suggests that insulin resistance is the common underlying cause of this syndrome. He postulates that insulin resistance and its compensatory hyperinsulinemia predisposes patients to hypertension, hyperlipidemia, and diabetes, and thus is the underlying cause of much CVD. Although obesity was not included in Reaven's primary list of disorders caused by insulin resistance, he acknowledged that obesity as well was correlated with insulin resistance or hyperinsulinemia. He suggests that a defect in insulin action plays a fundamental role in the development of the CVD risk factors that make up all definitions of the metabolic syndrome.

GLUCOSE INTOLERANCE

All three major diagnostic versions of the metabolic syndrome criteria include the requirement of some degree of abnormal glucose tolerance as reflected in the following criteria: abnormal glucose tolerance, elevated fasting glucose, type 2 diabetes, and elevated fasting insulin. This abnormality is most closely related to insulin resistance. It is now widely accepted that insulin resistance is a common characteristic of patients with type 2 diabetes, and that insulin resistance (or hyperinsulinemia as a surrogate estimate of insulin resistance) is a powerful and independent predictor of type 2 diabetes [5]. Also, the more severe the degree of insulin resistance, the higher the plasma glucose response to the oral glucose tolerance test [5]. Studies also show that even a minor degree of glucose intolerance in the nonobese individual is also associated with elevated blood pressure, dyslipidemic alterations (raised triacylglycerol and low HDL cholesterol), that form the remaining metabolic criteria of all three (WHO, ATP-III, IDF) definitions of the metabolic syndrome [3]. The lipoprotein abnormalities are part of the criteria of the WHO, the ATP-III, and the IDF, and are more likely to occur together and are significantly associated with insulin resistance and compensatory hyperinsulinemia. However, not all individuals with these abnormalities are insulin resistant. Insulin resistance or hyperinsulinemia is the only physiological abnormality that can result in the clustering of abnormalities that includes the atherogenic lipoprotein profile, in addition to elevated glucose level and elevated blood pressure [3].

Q: Is it justified to use the term metabolic syndrome?

The term *metabolic syndrome* is now widely accepted for this clinical condition, but there is still some discontent about its use. Some practitioners even question the very existence of this clinical condition. However, the ATP-III recommends using this term, and the NCEP introduced *metabolic syndrome* into the clinical guidelines for cholesterol-lowering therapy because of the recognition of the growing prevalence of risk-factor clustering in an increasingly obese population. The NCEP did acknowledge the importance of insulin resistance, but drew attention also to obesity, which contributes to this risk-factor clustering. Grundy [6] outlines the reasons for the NCEP's adopting the term *metabolic syndrome*. Metabolic risk factors commonly occur together. The concept of metabolic syndrome addresses the phenomenon of risk-factor clustering. This terminology enables a clinician to recognize that patients with a clustering of measured risk factors usually have several metabolic risk factors that are not readily apparent, for example, a prothrombotic state, a proinflammatory state, and multiple lipoprotein abnormalities including elevation of ApoB. The NCEP never intended the syndrome to be used as a predictor of short-term risk, and intended global risk assessment to be used instead for this purpose. Recognizing metabolic-risk factor clustering in practice is a way to identify patients who are at higher lifetime risk of CVD. These patients are also at increased lifetime risk of type 2 diabetes. The diagnosis of metabolic syndrome can be supportive of the global risk assessment in planning a therapeutic strategy for the patient.

Grundy address the dangers of taking literal meaning of words such as *aggressive* in the context of lipid-lowering therapy, and questioned the approach of treating each risk factor individually. For example, lifestyle interventions do no treat each factor individually but rather target multiple risk factors at once. The primary reason the NCEP introduced the metabolic syndrome into the clinical guidelines was to emphasize the importance of lifestyle therapy in clinical practice. Also, an effective therapeutic intervention will further enhance the treatment of multiple risk factors simultaneously.

The clinical diagnosis of the metabolic syndrome is useful because it affects the therapeutic strategy in patients at higher risk [7]. However, there are two views on the therapeutic strategy for patients with the metabolic syndrome. According to one view, each metabolic risk factor should be singled out and treated separately. The other view recommends that the therapeutic interventions should be aimed at reducing all the risk factors simultaneously. The latter approach emphasizes lifestyle interventions such as weight reduction and increased physical activity, which are aimed at all the risk factors. In fact, this approach also is the basis of other interventions for targeting multiple risk factors simultaneously by striking at the underlying cause.

Some drug therapies (e.g., nicotinic acid, fibrates) affect multiple risk factors simultaneously. The recommendation to treat each risk factor separately provides little guidance as to how best to treat the complex dyslipidemia of the metabolic syndrome. From the therapeutic angle, it would be more appropriate to use drugs that address the metabolic abnormalities as well, such as angiotensin-converting enzyme (ACE) inhibitors and ARBs (angiotensin receptor blockers) vs. thiazides and beta-blockers in antihypertensive therapy. In the future, there is hope of finding a drug that could affect multiple risk factors simultaneously.

Reaven [3] seems to believe that the term *metabolic syndrome* is not appropriate. He argues that because the diagnosis of the metabolic syndrome does not necessarily predict people at CVD risk, the purpose of diagnosis is completely lost, and it would then be clinically justified to treat each component of the metabolic syndrome per se. Reaven raises the question of whether a person's having the metabolic syndrome necessarily indicates that he or she is at greater risk of CVD than is a person who does not have the metabolic syndrome. A recent report from Framingham Study database [6] drew attention to the fact that a person having any two criteria of the metabolic syndrome was at no less risk than were those having three criteria. Reaven presents the clinical case of a 54-year-old man of European background with a WC of 93 cm, a plasma glucose of 203 mg/dL, and triglycerides of 193 mg/dL who does not have the metabolic syndrome according to the IDF criteria. If this individual is compared to another person who fulfills the IDF criteria of the metabolic syndrome, has a WC of 94 cm, a plasma glucose of 103 mg/dL, and triglycerides of 155 mg/dL, there is no doubt that the first patient has type 2 diabetes and a higher triglyceride level even though he is not eligible for the diagnosis of the metabolic syndrome, and is at greater CVD risk than the first. Similarly, there could be several other situations where the diagnosis of the metabolic syndrome is inappropriate and does not fulfill its obligatory prediction of CV risk

There are other problems with the definition of the metabolic syndrome: (1) The fact that there are several definitions confuses the clinician. (2) Statistics from studies are limited, especially from certain populations and for the young and the elderly. (3) The cutoff points for each feature of the syndrome are likely to differ among different populations in terms of the risk of diabetes or CVD. (4) The Framingham risk score is preferable over the metabolic syndrome in the risk assessment. (5) Such data are based on retrospective studies, and thus more prospective randomized trials are needed. (6) Some studies were small and any differences could be attributed to chance. (7) Not all studies address the problem of response rate, which could interfere with accurate estimation.

Q: What are the drawbacks with the various diagnostic criteria of the metabolic syndrome?

Kahn et al [7] addressed this issue very clearly in their paper. They drew attention to the fact that some of the criteria used for the definition of the metabolic syndrome are ambiguous or incomplete. The ATP-III seems to have modified some diagnostic criteria lately [2]; for example, the blood pressure requirement has changed from systolic ≥130 mm Hg/diastolic ≥85 mm Hg to ≥130 mm Hg *or* ≥85 mm Hg or on antihypertensive medication. The reason for this is not given. The guidelines on the measurement of blood pressure (i.e., supine, sitting, domiciliary reading) are not mentioned. It is also not clear if a patient who previously had an elevated IGF that now is normal after a weight loss should meet the criteria. These ambiguities can make differences in the diagnosis of some marginal cases, as only three of five criteria need to be fulfilled.

There are some marked differences between the WHO and the ATP-III criteria; for instance, the WHO has included microalbuminuria but the ATP-III has not. Additionally, the WHO has included insulin resistance (as measured under hyperinsulinemic-euglycemic conditions) but the ATP-III has not. The WHO also requires any evidence of insulin resistance, while the ATP-III is content with elevated fasting glucose. Kahn et al [7] suggest that the reasons for these differences in the criteria for the diagnosis need to be explained to medical practitioners to provide them with a better understanding. The original rationale of the criteria is that the components of the syndrome are associated with insulin resistance. If insulin resistance is the core of the syndrome, why not include age (arguably the most powerful predictor of insulin resistance)? There is also sufficient doubt about whether all individuals with the metabolic syndrome are insulin resistant. Kahn et al argue that the rationale of specific cutoff points, as opposed to higher and lower values, has never been delineated. Laaka et al [8] found that CVD and overall mortality in men with the metabolic syndrome was more consistently increased using a WC of 102 cm (as in the ATP-III) rather than 94 cm (the ethnicity-based criteria).

The WHO and ATP-III definitions are meant to identify same individuals, yet the National Health and Nutrition Examination Survey (NHANES-III) demonstrated the pitfalls of using these two criteria. Although approximately the same number were identified as having the syndrome by the WHO or ATP-III criteria (25% vs. 23.9% respectively), 15% to 20% of individuals were classified as having the syndrome by one criteria but not the other. The discrepancy in the number of cases of metabolic syndrome diagnosed with different definitions is discussed in Chapter 1. Kahn et al [7] suggest that the whole is not greater than the sum of its parts; therefore, the syndrome does not convey any additional risk beyond that of its components taken separately.

Because the risk factors cluster and because the CVD risk factors for the metabolic syndrome are linear in their damaging effect, different definitions of the metabolic syndrome make little difference in the prognostic implications. The features of the metabolic syndrome that are risk factors for CVD include (1) elevated plasma glucose level; (2) elevated blood pressure; (3) elevated serum triglycerides; (4) and low HDL cholesterol, as reflected in the plasma ApoB to ApoA ratios [9].

CARDIOVASCULAR DISEASE RISK AND THE METABOLIC SYNDROME

It is accepted that the metabolic syndrome is associated with increased prevalence of CVD, and this can be explained on the basis of that each individual component of the syndrome has been long known to be a major CVD risk factor. The ATP-III identified six components of the metabolic syndrome as "underlying," "major," and "emerging" CVD risk factors [1]. Kahn et al [7] suggested that there is ambiguity in the selection of the criteria. For instance, some risk factors associated with insulin resistance in each of the three categories (mentioned above) are not included. This is illustrated by the inclusion of obesity but not physical inactivity. Similarly, a family history, male gender, and advanced age, despite being major CVD risk factors, are excluded, but hypertension is included. Likewise, some emerging risk factors associated with insulin resistance, such as certain proinflammatory and prothrombotic markers, are not included, whereas raised triglycerides and glucose are. The ATP-III does not clarify why it includes only elevated triglycerides and glucose intolerance and excludes proinflammatory states and prothrombotic states from the criteria. There is substantial evidence that CRP is a strong independent predictor of a CV event and an independent marker of insulin resistance; its predictive value was equal to that of the metabolic syndrome [10]. The addition of CRP in the definition would have improved the diagnostic power. As discussed in the previous chapters, adipose tissue-derived cytokines (e.g., CRP, interleukin-6, tumor necrosis factor-α) and other markers (e.g., adiponectin) are linked to dyslipidemia, hypertension, and insulin action, which is why there is obvious interest in their predictive power of CVD risk. Adiponectin is not included in the diagnostic criteria by anyone, despite the evidence that it is consistently inversely related to insulin resistance, inflammation, and other CVD risk factors such as blood pressure, LDL cholesterol, and triglycerides. Likewise, plasminogen activator inhibitor-1 and fibrinogen are also inversely related but not included.

Another shortcoming is reflected in the equal weighting of each criterion in the ATP/WHO definition, yet it is well accepted that some components of the metabolic syndrome have higher CVD predictive value. In patients with the metabolic syndrome, the relative risk of CVD (or atherosclerotic cardiovascular disease) ranges from 1.5 to 3.0 depending on the stage of progression [11]. In the absence of diabetes, the risk of progression to type 2 diabetes ranges averages about a fivefold increase compared with those without the syndrome [11]. Once diabetes develops, the CVD risk increases even more. When diabetes exists concomitantly, the risk for subsequent CVD mortality is very high. If insulin resistance is at the core of the syndrome, why not include advanced age, as it is the most important predictor of insulin resistance. The fact that the metabolic syndrome as defined by the ATP-III is a relatively insensitive indicator of insulin resistance would seem to cast doubt on the fundamental premise that insulin resistance is optimally captured by the current definition [12]. Although the metabolic syndrome is supposed to identify patients with a higher long-term risk, none of the publications by the ATP-III mentioned that [12]. Moreover, a recent study of a cohort followed for 20 years found that the Framingham risk score was still a better CVD predictor tool than the metabolic syndrome [13]. Kahn et al disagree with Grundy's suggestion that the risk imparted by the condition is higher than the risk imparted by the component factors themselves. They further state that there is no clinical utility of the metabolic syndrome. Grundy argues that the clustering of five major risk factors of the metabolic syndrome cannot be explained by chance. Thus, if the metabolic syndrome is defined as multiple risk factors that are metabolically interrelated, then the syndrome exists.

References

1. Grundy SM, Brewer HB, Cleeman JI, et al. Criteria ATP-III: definition of metabolic syndrome. Circulation 2004;109:433–438.
2. Grundy SM, Cleeman JI, Daniels SR, et al. Diagnosis and management of the metabolic syndrome (AHA/NHLBI). Circulation 2005;112:2735–2752.
3. Reaven GM. The metabolic syndrome: is this diagnosis necessary? Am J Clin Nutr 2006;83:1237–1247.
4. Alberti KG, Zimmet PZ. Definition, diagnosis and classification of diabetes mellitus and its complications. Diabet Med 1998;15:539–553.
5. Reaven GM, Brand RJ, Chen Y-Di, et al. Insulin resistance and insulin secretion are determinants of oral glucose tolerance in normal individuals. Diabetes 1993;42:1224–1232.
6. Grundy SM. Does a diagnosis of metabolic syndrome have value in clinical practice? Am J Clin Nutr 2006;83:1248–1251.
7. Kahn R, Buse J, Ferrannini E, et al. The metabolic syndrome. Time for a critical appraisal. Diabetes Care 2005;28:2289–2304.
8. Laaka H-M, Laaksonen DE, Lakka TA, et al. The metabolic syndrome and total and CVD mortality in middle-aged men. JAMA 2002;288:2709–2716.

9. Hanley AJ, Karter AJ, Williams K, et al. Predictor of type 2 diabetes with alternative definitions of the metabolic syndrome. Circulation 2005;112:3713–3721.
10. Ridker PM, Buring JE, Cook NR, et al. CRP metabolic syndrome and risk of CV events. Circulation 2003;107:391–397.
11. Grundy SM. Metabolic syndrome: connecting and reconciling CV and diabetes world. J Am Coll Cardiol 2006;47:1093–1100.
12. Kahn R. The metabolic syndrome (Emperor) wears no clothes. Diabetic Care 2006;29:1693–1695.
13. Wannamethee SG, Sharper AG, Lennon L, et al. Metabolic syndrome vs. Framingham risk score for prevention of CHD, stroke and type 2 diabetes. Arch Intern Med 2005;165:2644–2650.

Chapter 5
Consequences of the
Metabolic Syndrome

CARDIOVASCULAR DISEASE AND DIABETES

Q: What is the evidence that metabolic syndrome and its components affect the development of cardiovascular disease and type 2 diabetes? Various recent studies have described the association among the metabolic syndrome, diabetes, and cardiovascular disease (CVD) morbidity and mortality (including all-cause mortality where applicable). The findings may vary with the diagnostic criteria used. The relative risk of the metabolic syndrome was generally highest for coronary heart disease (CHD) mortality, intermediate for CVD mortality, and lowest (and not necessarily statistically significant) for all-cause mortality [1]. Because the prevalence of the metabolic syndrome is increasing alarmingly among adolescents and young adults, it is important to quantify its relation with clinical coronary artery disease (CAD) occurring early in life.

The metabolic syndrome is associated with an increased risk of CVD and diabetes [2] as well as a major contributor to long-term morbidity and cost. The risk of incident CHD or fatal CHD is two to four times higher in diabetics than in nondiabetics. Most individuals who develop CVD have multiple risk factors. Most individuals with the metabolic syndrome have insulin resistance, which confers an increased risk of type 2 diabetes. Studies have found that the CVD risk in patients with the syndrome ranged from 30% to 300%; this wide variation is probably due to population studies, the precise definition used, and the length of follow-up. Three studies have assessed whether the difference in prevalence between the two definitions affects the predictive power for subsequent CVD [2, 3, 60]. Two of these studies found the Adult Treatment Panel (ATP-III) to be a slightly better predictor of the all-cause and cardiovascular (CV) mortality [3, 60], whereas one study found that the World Health Organization (WHO) definition more consistently predicted CVD and all-cause mortality [2]. In the San Antonio Study there were

2815 participants aged 25 to 64 years. In the general population, the all-cause mortality hazard ratio (HRs) were 1.47 (95% confidence interval (CI), 1.13–1.92) for the National Cholesterol Education Program (NCEP) metabolic syndrome, and 1.27 (95% CI, 0.97–1.66) for WHO-Mets. Furthermore, for CV mortality, there was evidence that gender modified the predictive ability of the M. S. For women & men, respectively, HRs for NCEP-Mets were 4.65 (95% CI, 2.35–9.21) and 1.82 (95% CI, 1.14–2.91), whereas HRs for the WHO metabolic syndrome the HRs were 2.83 (95% CI, 1.55–5.17) and 1.15 (95% CI, 0.72–1.86). The study concluded that the NCEP definition tended to be more predictive in lower-risk patients [3].

Some risk factors associated with insulin resistance were not included in this study, such as physical activity. It has been suggested that if other risk factors are included in the definition, the predictive value of the syndrome will improve. However, no study has examined the impact of this definition. Also, the issue of whether the risk factors act synergistically has not been resolved. Nevertheless, C-reactive protein (CRP) has been found to be an independent CVD risk factor and independent marker of insulin resistance.

Most individuals who develop the metabolic syndrome first acquire abdominal obesity without risk factors, but with time, multiple risk factors appear. Epidemiological studies suggest that multiple risk factors increase the risk more than the sum of the accompanying single risk factors; the risk rises geometrically instead of linearly. This phenomenon is called multiplicative risk [4]. Obesity and physical inactivity independently contribute to the development of CHD in women [5].

In the San Antonio Study, the relative risk of diabetes is at least threefold greater among individuals with the metabolic syndrome, though the diagnostic criteria taken into account do affect the risk. The relative risk using the ATP-III criteria is 3.30 (2.27–4.80) [6]. The presence of the metabolic syndrome is a significant predictor for CVD and type 2 diabetes, but a stronger predictor for type 2 diabetes than of CHD. Although the metabolic syndrome does not predict CHD as well as the Framingham risk score (FRS), it serves well as a single clinical tool for identifying high-risk subjects predisposed to CVD or type 2 diabetes (San Antonio Heart Study) [6]. The above study shows that impaired glucose tolerance (IGT) and the NCEP definition of the metabolic syndrome have comparable sensitivity for predicting diabetes. However, the IGT had a higher positive predictor value than each of the definitions of the metabolic syndrome. Impaired glucose tolerance and impaired fasting glucose (IFG) are both strong predictors of diabetes. The oral glucose tolerance test identifies more high-risk subjects than does

IFG. The metabolic syndrome is not better than IGT for detecting subjects at high risk for diabetes. However, the combination of IGT and the NCEP definition detects 70% of subjects at high risk for diabetes [6].

A disproportionate impact of glucose intolerance (IFG/IGT/-diabetes) in the syndrome definition was demonstrated by Malik et al [7] in their study of National Health and Nutrition Examination Survey (NHANES-II) participants. They observed that diabetes alone conveyed a much greater risk of CHD (HR = 5), CVD, or overall mortality than the presence of the metabolic syndrome (3.5, 2.7, and 1.5, respectively), according to definitions that included individuals with and without IFG/IGT/diabetes. Adding preexisting CVD to diabetes was an even more powerful predictor of mortality (11.3, 7.9, and 2.9, respectively) over the 13-year follow-up period. Additionally, Hunt et al [3] also showed that the presence of IFG (>6.1 mmol/L [110 mg/L]) alone was a stronger predictor of CVD or all-cause mortality in the general population than either the syndrome as a whole or any of its individual components. Interestingly, this finding raises questions of why glucose intolerance (particularly diabetes) is included in the definition of the metabolic syndrome, since it appears to account for most, if not all, of the CVD predictive value.

The metabolic syndrome is associated with a threefold increase in the likelihood of death from CHD [4]. In the European study [2] and in the Verona Diabetes Complication Study [8], the relative hazard ratio for CVD outcomes ranged from 2 to 5. The metabolic syndrome is significantly associated with myocardial infarction (MI) and stroke, and therefore it has clinical utility in identifying patients at increased risk of MI and the metabolic syndrome [9]. Also, applying the ATP-III criteria to 10,357 NHANES-III participants led to a significant association between the metabolic syndrome and MI and stroke [9]. In this study the metabolic syndrome was significantly related in multivariate analysis to MI (odds ratio [OR], 2.01; 95% CI, 1.53–2.64), stroke (OR, 2.16; 95% CI, 1.48–3.16), and MI/stroke (OR, 2.05; 95% CI, 1.64–2.57). The syndrome was significantly associated with MI/stroke in both women and men. Among the component conditions, insulin resistance (OR, 1.30; 95% CI, 1.03–1.66), low high-density lipoprotein (HDL) cholesterol (OR, 1.35; 95% CI, 1.05–1.74), hypertension (OR, 1.44; 95% CI, 1.00–2.08), and hypertriglyceridemia (OR, 1.66; 95% CI, 1.20–2.30) were independently and significantly related to MI/stroke [9]. Finally, this study found that with the exception of waist circumference, all of the components of the metabolic syndrome were significantly associated with MI/stroke. Moreover, the risk of CVD and diabetes increases as the number of components of the metabolic syndrome increase [10]. In the Diabetes Epidemiology Collaborative Analysis of Diagnostic Criteria in Europe (DECODE) study involving European men and women, nondiabetic individuals with the metabolic syndrome had an increased risk of death from all causes as well as from CVD [11]. The overall prevalence of the metabolic syndrome in nondiabetic adults in Europe is 15%. The overall hazard ratios for all-cause and CVD mortality in people with the metabolic syndrome compared with those without it were 1.44 and 2.26 for men and 1.38 and 2.78 for women after adjustment for age, blood cholesterol level, and smoking [11].

Lakka et al [12] found a 3.2 relative risk of acute coronary events in individuals with features of the metabolic syndrome (body mass index [BMI] ≥ 25.0 and waist/hip ratio ≥ 0.91). In the Women's Angiographic Vitamin and Estrogen Trial, the prevalence of the metabolic syndrome was 60%, and clinical CV events were significantly more frequent in those without the metabolic syndrome [13]. Ridker et al [14] found that patients with the metabolic syndrome are at increase risk of type 2 diabetes (sevenfold higher) and a CVD event (70% to 200% higher). Once diabetes develops, the CV risk increases further.

In a cross-sectional data analysis from the NHANES-III population, the prevalence of CHD was increased with the metabolic syndrome (WHO criteria) [15]; 86% of individuals over the age of 50 years living in the United States who have type 2 diabetes qualify for the diagnosis of metabolic syndrome [15]. Individuals over 50 years of age without the metabolic syndrome had the lowest CHD prevalence, and this was similar regardless of diabetes status (8.7% among nondiabetics, 7.5% among individuals with diabetes). In the absence of diabetes, the metabolic syndrome was associated with CHD prevalence of 13.9%, while in the presence of diabetes the prevalence increases to 19.2%. The association of the metabolic syndrome with the prevalence of CHD is not independent of blood pressure, HDL cholesterol, and diabetes [15].

The presence of the metabolic syndrome at the time of the diagnosis of diabetes was an independent predictor of incident CVD during 5 years of follow-up [16]. There was a linear increase in incident cardiovascular risk with an increasing number of features of the metabolic syndrome present at the time of diagnosis of type 2 diabetes. With the presence of all five features, there was an almost fivefold increase as compared with hyperglycemia alone. The ATP-III criteria were superior to the WHO criteria in the San Antonio study, but the WHO criteria better predicted CVD in Finnish men.

The concept of a syndrome implies that the risk associated with the syndrome ought to be greater than the risk associated with its parts. In a recent study, after adjusting for external risk factors, the presence of the metabolic syndrome by the ATP-III criteria in the absence of diabetes conferred an almost fivefold increase in the odds of early-onset CAD; combined with diabetes, the odds ratio was 8 (early onset included acute MI [AMI], angina with confirmed angiographic stenosis >50%, and revascularization procedures). The American Heart Association (AHA)/National Heart, Lung, and Blood Institute (NHLBI) definition resulted in a slightly better prediction of outcome: the odds ratio was almost 6 and 10, respectively, for the metabolic syndrome without diabetes and with diabetes. However, in multivariate analysis, the metabolic syndrome (regardless of the definition used) conveyed no additional predictive information beyond its components, casting doubt on its clinical utility [17]. Previous investigators have reached similar conclusions. For instance, blood pressure (BP), HDL cholesterol, and diabetes, but not the presence of the metabolic syndrome, were significant multivariate predictors of the prevalence of CHD in the recent analysis of the NHANES-III.

The Framingham Heart Study followed a cohort of 3323 middle-aged adults for development of new CVD, CHD, and type 2 diabetes. Over an 8-year period, in persons without CVD or type 2 diabetes at baseline, the prevalence of the metabolic syndrome (at least three of the five criteria) was 26.8% in men and 16.6% in women. Wilson et al [18] found that the population-attributable risk estimates associated with the metabolic syndrome for CVD, CHD, and type 2 diabetes were 34%, 29%, and 62%, respectively, in men and 16%, 8%, 47%, respectively, in women [18]. The metabolic syndrome was associated with an increased risk for CVD and type 2 diabetes for both sexes. The metabolic syndrome accounted for up to one third (relative risk [RR], 2.88; 95% CI, 1.99–4.16; PAR (population-attributable risk), 33.7%) of CVD in men and approximately half (RR, 6.92; 95% CI, 4.47–10.81; PAR, 61.5%) of new type 2 diabetes over 8 years' follow-up. In women, the corresponding figures for CVD are RR, 2.25; 95% CI, 1.31–3.88; PAR, 15.8%; and for diabetes, RR, 6.90; 95% CI, 4.35–10.94; PAR, 46.9%. Wilson et al provide clear evidence that insulin resistance and its cluster of associated abnormalities increase the risk of type 2 diabetes and CVD. They also emphasize that the cluster of abnormalities related to insulin resistance are more powerful predictors of type 2 diabetes than of CVD, presumably because there certainly are CVD risk factors unrelated to insulin resistance, for example, elevated low-density lipoprotein cholesterol. The two best predictors of adverse CVD outcomes in this study were elevated blood pressure and a low HDL cholesterol, whereas the best predictor of type 2 diabetes was the fasting plasma glucose.

In the Framingham study, the metabolic syndrome alone predicted 25% of all new-onset CVD. In the absence of diabetes, the metabolic syndrome did not raise the 10-year risk to >20%. The 10-year risk in men with the metabolic syndrome rose from 10% to 20%. Women participants had fewer CHD events during the period of study. The 10-year CHD risk in this young group of women remained less than 10%. The Framingham data showed that most men with diabetes had a 10-year risk of CHD >20%; in contrast, women rarely exceed the 20% level. The Framingham Offspring Study [18] showed that compared with normal glucose tolerance (NGT), individuals with IFG/IGT were more likely (diabetics significantly more) to have subclinical coronary atherosclerosis. Individuals with previously diagnosed metabolic syndrome had a three times greater risk than those recently diagnosed based on IGT. Individuals with insulin resistance were twice as likely to have subclinical coronary atherosclerosis as those without insulin resistance. However, this association became diluted when adjusted for other risk factors such as cigarette smoking, total cholesterol/HDL cholesterol ratio, and systolic blood pressure.

A systemic review and meta-analysis of 37 eligible longitudinal studies found that the metabolic syndrome had a relative risk (RR) of CVD events and death of 1.78 (95% CI, 1.58–2.00) [19]. The association was stronger in women (RR, 2.63 vs. 1.98, $p = .09$), in studies enrolling lower risk (<10%) individuals (RR, 1.96 vs. 1.43, $p = .04$), and in studies using factor analysis or the WHO definition (RR, 2.68 or 2.06, vs. 1.67 for the NCEP definition and 1.35 for another definition, $p = .005$). The association remained after adjusting for traditional CV risk factors. The best available evidence suggests that people with the metabolic syndrome are at increased risk of CV events. The data demonstrated that the CV risk confirmed by the metabolic syndrome was a third higher in women.

EXCESS ADIPOSITY

Q: What are the effects of different components of the metabolic syndrome on cardiovascular disease?
Unlike dyslipidemia, hyperglycemia, and hypertension (other components of the metabolic syndrome), adiposity does not directly increase the CVD risk and therefore has a different relationship with the metabolic syndrome. The components of the metabolic syndrome occur more commonly in overweight or obese individuals, but this relationship is not due to obesity per se, but rather to the fact

that excess adiposity increases the likelihood that an individual will be insulin resistant [19]. Moreover, the data from the NHANES-III also showed that obesity (ATP-III criteria) was the only criterion not statistically associated with the development of either CVD or stroke [20]. The authors reasoned that the findings may reflect an indirect effect of increased waist circumference (WC) through other components of the syndrome. However, the European Group for the Study of Insulin Resistance (EGIR) found that only 25% of obese volunteers were classified as being insulin-resistant according to the criteria used. The EGIR also clarified that the differences it noted in WC were unrelated to insulin sensitivity after adjustment for age, sex, and BMI [21]. Though BMI and WC are highly correlated, WC does not automatically qualify as the superior predictor of the adverse effect of excess obesity. This is supported by the findings in NHANES-III, which showed that the coefficient between BMI and WC was >0.9 irrespective of age, sex, or ethnicity [22]. Because the relationship between insulin-mediated glucose uptake (IMGU) and overall obesity (BMI) does not differ significantly from that between IMGU and abdominal obesity (WC), it seems that either index of adiposity is equally predictive of differences in insulin action.

The landmark Framingham study showed that in men and women aged 49 to 82 years, the most important risk factor for CHD was low HDL cholesterol, which was found to be an independent predictor of CHD risk, even when LDL cholesterol levels were low [23]. The association between risk factors and mortality from CHD was also investigated by the Multiple Risk Factor Intervention Trial (MRFIT) research group, which found that age, diastolic blood pressure, cigarette smoking, LDL cholesterol, and HDL cholesterol were all significant risk factors [24]. The Prospective Cardiovascular Munster (PROCAM) study further confirmed the significant association between CHD and HDL cholesterol, with data indicating triglycerides as a powerful additional coronary risk factor [25]. The risk of CAD was found to be nearly doubled if triglyceride levels were ≥ 2.2 mmol/L or the HDL cholesterol level was <1 mmol/L; with both these risk factors present, there was a fourfold increase in risk. There was a strong link between increasing CAD risk and decreasing levels of HDL cholesterol at all levels of triglycerides [26].

Each component of the metabolic syndrome is a risk factor of CVD, and the combination of even moderate levels of the risk factors has a synergistic effect. Even though the prevalence of CVD is declining, the increased incidence of type 2 diabetes may reverse this trend in the future. Dyslipidemia is an established independent risk factor for CVD. Low HDL cholesterol and hypertriglyceridemia have been noted to be significantly and independently related to MI/stroke in individuals with the metabolic syndrome. Also, a combination of high fasting glucose and low HDL cholesterol are shown to be a primary predictor of CHD. Components of the metabolic syndrome are associated with an incident CVD and diabetes after 5 years. These components are reported to precede the detection of overt diabetes by as much as 10 years, at which time the known increased risk of CVD has been documented, but smoking, alcohol intake, and physical inactivity may further modify the risk [27]. Klein et al [27] studied the relationship of CVD and diabetes to the components of the metabolic syndrome. In their study they used the WHO criteria of diagnosis of the metabolic syndrome. They found that components of the metabolic syndrome singly and in combination are common and precede incident CVD and diabetes [27] (Table 5.1).

In clinical practice a pragmatic approach might be to treat the components of the metabolic syndrome, such as BMI, blood pressure, and lipids, early on to reduce the incidence of CHD and diabetes. Reducing even one or two of the components of the metabolic syndrome may reduce the overall risk of incident CVD and diabetes. As the correlation between the components is significant, treatment of one component may have an effect on the others. Therefore, decreasing the BMI may have a beneficial effect on blood pressure, lipid level, and uric acid level. Treating the hypertension may have a good effect on the kidney, at least with respect to microalbuminuria. An elevated serum triglyceride level represents an independent risk factor for CHD, especially in women.

TABLE 5.1. The incidence of cardiovascular disease (CVD) and diabetes by components of the metabolic syndrome

Components	% Incidence of CVD		% Incidence of diabetes	
	Normal level	Elevated level	Normal level	Elevated level
Elevated glycemia	5.5	14.1	2.0	29.1
High blood pressure	5.8	6.7	3.2	5.2
High-risk lipid levels	3.4	6.5	2.4	3.7
Elevated BMI	5.6	6.7	1.9	6.7
Elevated uric acid	4.8	9.5	2.7	5.9
Proteinuria	5.8	12.9	3.5	3.7

Source: Klein et al. [27].

Endothelial Dysfunction

Endothelial dysfunction predisposes to atherosclerosis in the presence of increased prothrombotic factors such as coagulation abnormalities, increase platelet activation, inflammatory mediators, and the presence of oxidized lipoproteins. Endothelial dysfunction is not only a critical event in the subsequent development of CV complications of diabetes but also precedes the clinically detectable plaque in coronary disease and serves as a pivotal event in the atherosclerosis.

Hyperinsulinemia/Insulin Resistance

Hyperinsulinemia or insulin resistance is associated with the development of CVD, but the exact mechanism is uncertain. A recent study reaffirmed the significant independent association of CVD mortality with both fasting hyperinsulinemia and a homeostasis model of insulin resistance [11]. This study had the limitation of a paucity of measurements of insulin resistance. However, another prospective study that did measure insulin resistance confirmed that insulin resistance predicts the CVD risk [28]. The CV mortality was increased in both Hispanics and non-Hispanics. Of the proinflammatory factors, CRP has drawn considerable attention, but the white cell count appears to have closer relationship to CHD. The higher the white cell count, the greater the insulin resistance, and the greater the plasma glucose and insulin response to oral glucose challenge, the higher the triglycerides and the lower the HDL cholesterol.

Procoagulant, Leptin, and Adiponectin

Factor VII activity is increased during postprandial hyperlipidemia, predisposing an individual to an acute CAD event after consumption of a high-fat meal. Plasminogen activator inhibitor-1 (PAI-1) is known to be a marker of premature CVD. Hyperinsulinemia may also directly inhibit fibrinolysis in individuals with insulin resistance. Low plasma levels have been associated with the progression of coronary artery calcification in type 1 diabetics and nondiabetics, independent of other CVD risk factors.

Q: How does particle size increase CV risk?

Small, dense LDL particles are associated with a threefold increase in the CHD risk. This finding is supported by the Quebec Cardiovascular Study, in which men with an LDL particle size < 25.6 nm had a significant 2.2-fold increase in the 5-year rate of ischemic heart disease (IHD) compared with men who had LDL particle size > 25.6 nm [29]. A subgroup analysis further emphasized that the risk posed by the LDL small particle size was independent of LDL cholesterol, HDL cholesterol, apolipoprotein B (ApoB), triglycerides, and the total cholesterol/HDL cholesterol ratio. These findings, however, were refuted by the Physicians' Health Study, in which LDL particle size was no longer a statistically significant risk factor, but triglycerides and total cholesterol (not HDL cholesterol) were [30]. Subclasses of very low density lipoprotein (VLDL), LDL, and HDL were also studied by proton nuclear magnetic resonance (NMR) spectroscopy, to determine if their variation had implications in CVD prediction rate [31]. This study suggested that CAD risk was positively associated with levels of large VLDL and small HDL particles, and inversely with a high number of intermediate-size HDL particles. Men with high levels of small HDL or large VLDL particle size were at three- to fourfold greater risk of extensive CAD as compared to men with lower levels. Furthermore, coexistence of both large VLDL and small HDL in the same man increases the risk to 15-fold. It has been suggested that the size of LDL particle size and number of LDL particles are related to incident CHD among women.

In the Apoliprotein-Related Mortality Risk (AMORIS) Study, ApoB and the ApoB/ApoA-I ratio have also been suggested to be associated with increased risk of future MI in both men and women [32]. Although hypertriglyceridemia has been found to be an independent risk factor for CVD, it is possible that it may not be elevated triglyceride per se that is atherogenic but instead it is a marker for increased triglyceride-rich remnant lipoprotein, which in turn is associated with the atherosclerotic disease [33]. There is an inverse relationship between the size of lipoproteins and their ability to cross the endothelial barrier to pass through the arterial intima to enter the subendothelial space. Chylomicrons and large VLDLs (Svedbery flotation unit [S_1] 60–400) are probably not able to enter the arterial wall, whereas small VLDLs (S_1 20 to 60) and intermediate-density lipoproteins (IDLs) (S_1 12 to 20) are capable and were independently correlated with the development of coronary atherosclerosis. This explains why some triglycerides are atherogenic whereas others are not. Furthermore, triglyceride-rich lipoproteins (such as VLDLs and particles rich in ApoC-III) were related to the progression of mild to moderate (< 50% diameter stenosis), coronary artery lesions rather than severe (≥50% diameter stenosis) lesions [34]. Remnant-like particles (RLPs), that is, RLP cholesterol and RLP triglycerides, are highly increased in diabetic women and diabetic men compared with controls. ApoC-III in VLDL is associated with denser, small LDL subclasses that have greater atherogenicity; likewise, remnants associated with ApoC-III are more atherogenic than triglycerides per se.

Triglyceride-rich Remnant Lipoprotein

There is direct relationship between (small size) VLDL/LDL and atherogenism. Remnant lipoproteins derived from chylomicrons or VLDL (i.e., lipoprotein subclasses LP-B:C, LP-B:C:E, and Lp-A-11:B: C:D:L) enhance atherogenesis. Studies show that VLDL cholesterol, VLDL-triglyceride, VLDL-ApoB, ApoC-III, and ApoE in HDL all predicted subsequent coronary events in the Cholesterol and Recurrent Events (CARE) [35]. The VLDL particles and ApoC-III in VLDL and LDL more reliably predicted CHD risk than did plasma triglycerides. In the Framingham Offspring Study, both RLPs (RLP cholesterol) and RLP-triglycerides were appreciably increased in women with diabetes ($p < .0001$) and men ($p < .0001$) compared with control nondiabetics [36].

NONALCOHOLIC FATTY LIVER DISEASE

Q: What features do fatty liver disease share with the metabolic syndrome, and what are its clinical implications?

Nonalcoholic fatty liver disease (NAFLD) is emerging as a component of the metabolic syndrome because of its close association with other features of the syndrome, such as obesity, central obesity, diabetes, dyslipidemia, hypertension, and atherosclerotic CVD. Its severity is directly proportional to the severity of insulin resistance. Nonalcoholic steatohepatitis (NASH), though uncommon as recently as 3 years ago, is becoming quite common in the U.S. Recently, the liver has been recognized as a major target of injury in patients with insulin resistance or the metabolic syndrome. Insulin resistance is associated with fat accumulation in the liver, a condition termed nonalcoholic fatty liver disease. Excess fat in the liver is not a benign condition. Some patients with NAFLD develop necroinflammatory changes in the liver, termed nonalcoholic steatohepatitis, and a fraction of those patients will develop cirrhosis. About 20% of all adults have NAFLD and 2% to 3% of adults have NASH [37].

In NASH triglyceride accumulation and inflammation coexist. There are many causes of abnormal liver functions, but a growing number of individuals are found to have NASH, which is a disorder with histological features of alcohol-induced liver disease in the absence of alcohol. Nonalcoholic fatty liver disease is associated with severe obesity and a BMI of >35. For descriptive purpose, NASH and NAFLD will be collectively defined as NASH. Hyperglycemia and hyperlipidemia are common associations that are thought to be predisposing this condition.

Conditions commonly associated with fatty liver are obesity (70% to 100% are obese), hypertension, diabetes/insulin resistance, and hyperlipidemia, such as abetalipoproteinemia and hypolipoproteinemia. Some patients are lean, have normal fasting glucose and normal glucose tolerance, and manifest no evidence of increased plasma lipids, but 85% of individuals have the metabolic syndrome/insulin resistance and 70% have a family history of diabetes mellitus. Other factors that may contribute to fatty liver are certain drugs (aspirin, glucocorticoids, synthetic estrogen, tetracycline, methotrexate), environmental toxins, atherosclerotic disease, total parenteral nutrition, and jejunoileal or gastric bypass. Fatty liver may worsen other existing liver conditions such as hepatitis C. Nonalcoholic steatohepatitis is more preventable than hepatitis C, hepatitis B, and alcoholic liver disease.

It is not as yet clear whether markers of NAFLD, including elevated concentrations of aspartate aminotransferase (AST), alanine aminotransferase (ALT), and alkaline phosphatase, predict the development of metabolic syndrome. The concentrations of ALT and the AST/ALT ratio are positively associated with the risk of developing the metabolic syndrome after adjustment of covariants, including demographic variables, alcoholic intake, abdominal obesity, and IGT. The increase in ALT and γ-glutamyltransferase (γ-GT) is less marked than in alcoholic liver disease. Independent predictors of NASH and advanced pericellular fibrosis are ALT greater than normal, hypertension, and either insulin resistance index (NASH) or fasting C-peptide (fibrosis) [38]. Typically, fatty liver is associated with serum AST and serum ALT values >250 U/L or modest elevation of serum alkaline phosphatase. Serum ALT or AST values >300 U/L usually suggest an alternative pathology. An AST/ALT ratio >2 is suggestive of alcohol liver disease. Half of patients have raised serum ferritin. The condition is asymptomatic, but some patients may complain of discomfort in the right upper quadrant, malaise, or fatigue, and examination may reveal hepatomegaly. In children acanthosis nigricans may be present with NAFLD.

Ultrasonography is the most popular imaging modality for the diagnosis of NAFLD, but computed tomography (CT) and magnetic resonance imaging (MRI) are more sensitive. However, liver biopsy remains the gold standard. The distinction between NAFLD and NASH are only made by histology and cannot be predicted by clinical or laboratory investigation. From a clinical point of view, a few patients have ongoing liver injury; 50% of NASH patients develop liver fibrosis, 15% develop cirrhosis, and 3% may progress to terminal liver failure requiring liver transplantation. If liver enzymes are persistently raised, liver biopsy is indicated.

Pathogenesis

Insulin Resistance

The exact mechanism of NASH is not clear. However, insulin resistance and hyperinsulinemia play key roles [39]. Marchesini et al [39] reported that, using the homeostasis model assessment (HOMA) method, insulin resistance was the laboratory finding most closely associated with the presence of NAFLD in a large series of patients, irrespective of BMI, fat distribution, or glucose tolerance. Therefore, NAFLD might represent another feature of the metabolic syndrome. Day [38] proposed a "two-hit hypothesis," with lipids acting as the first hit and increased lipid peroxide being the second hit. The first hit, steatosis, sensitizes the liver to the second hit, which leads to microinflammation and fibrosis [38]. The principal target for first hit are both peripheral and hepatic insulin resistance while oxidative stress and abnormal cytokine production are second hit. Insulin resistance may be both first and second hit.

Besides insulin resistance, oxidative stress and abnormal cytokine production are the principal etiological factors. There remain unknown genetic and acquired factors (e.g., central obesity) responsible for insulin resistance, which leads to the development of steatosis through increased lipolysis and delivery of free fatty acids (FFAs) to the liver. A primary role for insulin resistance is supported by the high frequency of steatosis in inherited syndromes of severe insulin resistance and amelioration of steatosis in the *ob/ob* leptin-deficient mouse model of steatosis with metformin, which improves hepatic insulin resistance [38]. An abnormal cytokine production seems to be due to (1) an abnormal macrophage function; (2) an effect of oxidative stress through nuclear translocation of transcription nuclear factor (NF)-κB and direct release by adipose tissue (e.g., tumor necrosis factor-α [TNF-α]); or (3) bacterial overgrowth [38].

Resistance to the antilipolytic action of insulin in adipose tissue results in increase FFA flux to the liver. In the liver there is also increased production of nonesterified fatty acids (NEFAs) from glucose not taken up by peripheral adipocytes and monocytes. As not all FFAs are oxidized, some are converted to diacyl- and triacylglycerols and stored in the hepatic cytoplasm, leading to steatosis. This effect is further aggravated by insulin resistance affecting the activity of peroxisome proliferator-activated receptors α and γ (PPARα and PPARγ) and sterol regulatory element-binding proteins (SREBPs) [1]. It is probable that a metabolite of lipid breakdown initiated through lipid peroxide generation triggers the inflammatory response and increased NF-κB activity that contributes to cellular activation and further cytokine release [1].

Recently, the role of the rennin-angiotensin system in promoting insulin resistance has been observed. Endoplasmic reticulum (ER) stress has also become a recent target of investigation because ER stress is common in obesity, diabetes, and various forms of liver disease including NAFLD. Endoplasmic reticulum stress may be responsible for the activation of c-Jun kinase, a process that may cause the hepatocellular injury in NASH. Progress has also been made in estimating the prevalence of NAFLD in adults and children. Patients enrolled in the Dallas Heart Study were found to have a 33% prevalence of NAFLD, and children dying in accidents in San Diego were found to have a 13% prevalence of NAFLD. Because about 10% of people with NAFLD are at risk for progressive fibrosis, the burden of disease is now quite substantial [40].

Obesity

Overexpression of TNF-α by adipose tissue has been suggested to play role in the development of NASH, linking NASH with obesity and type 2 diabetes. Rad is also implicated in the pathogenesis of NASH. It is a member of the RGK (Rem, Rad, Gem and Kir) family of Ras-related guanosine triphosphatases (GTPases) and leptin. Its overexpression in skeletal muscle in type 2 diabetes interferes with cell function and is thus linked to insulin resistance. Leptin exerts its effect in insulin resistance and NASH through dephosphorylation of insulin receptor substrate-1 (IRS-1).

Oxidative Stress

Mitochondria are the main cellular source of reactive oxygen species (ROS), which may initiate the inflammatory component of NASH. Oxidative stress plays an important role in the pathogenesis of NASH [41]. The cytochrome P-450 enzymes CYP2E1 and CYP4A are able to generate free radicals to enhance oxidative stress. Both enzymes regulate the hydroxylation of fatty acid and the production of lipid peroxide. The production of lipid peroxide is increased when these enzymes are upregulated [42]. CYP2E1 has been observed to be upregulated persistently in type 2 diabetes, insulin resistance, visceral obesity, and NASH, and CYP2E1 also is upregulated by a high-fat/low-carbohydrate diet. When levels of glutathione are reduced, the toxicity of arachidonic acid in CYP2E1-overexpressing cells is increased [42]. Overexpression of CYP2E1 suggests an important role for antioxidants in preventing hepatocyte injury in NASH. Additionally, CYP2E1 also may induce hepatic fibrosis.

Adiponectin appears to have a hepatoprotective effect, and a direct antiinflammatory effect through TNF-α. Experiment studies show that adiponectin is effective in reducing hepatomegaly, steatosis, and serum ALT levels in obese animals [43]. This indicates that adiponectin may act directly or indirectly in influencing the incriminating factor for NASH.

Sterol Regulatory Element-binding Proteins
Sterol regulatory element-binding proteins (SREBPs) are a family of regulated transcription factors that stimulate lipid synthesis in the liver. They induce the expression of more than 30 genes involved in the synthesis and uptake of cholesterol, fatty acids, triacylglycerols, and phospholipids, and the NADPH required to synthesize these lipids. To date, three SREBP isoforms have been identified and characterized. SREBP-1a and -1c are derived from a single gene and SREBP-2 from a separate gene. In the liver they regulate the production of lipid export into the plasma as lipoproteins and into the bile as micelles. Expression of SREBP-1c in the liver increases fatty acid synthesis and may also contribute to the regulation of glucose uptake and glucose synthesis. The SREBP-1c levels are increased in the fatty livers of obese *(ob/ob)* mice with insulin resistance and hyperinsulinemia caused by leptin deficiency, and SREBP-1c increases lipogenic gene expression, increases fatty acid synthesis, and accelerates triacylglycerol accumulation [44]. Leptin administration opposes SREBP-1c levels and reverses these metabolic derangements [44]. Metformin decreases hepatic SREBP-1 levels and lowers lipid accumulation in the liver of insulin-resistant *ob/ob* mice [45]. These studies support the idea that elevated SREBP-1c levels cause the fatty liver seen in insulin resistance. Overexpression of SREBP-1a in rats resulted in a 26-fold increase in fatty acid synthesis and a fivefold increase in cholesterol synthesis, and SREBP-2 overexpression in transgenic mice caused a 28-fold increase in cholesterol synthesis and a fourfold increase in fatty acid synthesis. These data from these studies support the idea that SREBP-1a, SREBP-1c, and SREBP-2 play a role in the pathogenesis of NASH.

Role of Pharmacological Agents
There are no specific long-term recommendations, but the treatment with PPARα and PPARγ agonists, biguanides, antioxidant therapy (vitamin E), and ursodeoxycholic acid as well as physical exercise and weight loss in obese subjects are important. Administration of the PPARγ agonist rosiglitazone for 24 weeks in 30 individuals with NASH improved insulin sensitivity, reduced liver fat content, and improved the biochemical evidence (ALT level) of hepatocellular injury [46]. Besides improving insulin sensitivity, it is likely that part of the benefit may have been due to antiinflammatory effect of the PPARγ ligand.

It is not proven as yet if metformin has a definite role in the treatment of NASH. However, results of some recent studies are encouraging. In one study, 36 patients with NASH were treated with metformin for 6 months [47]. The liver enzymes and C-peptide levels decreased, and the index of insulin resistance also markedly improved. But no significant differences in necroinflammatory activity or fibrosis were observed. The metformin-treated group showed a trend toward improved hepatic necroinflammatory activity, with decreased steatosis, ballooning of hepatocytes, and acinar portal inflammation. Histological lesions of steatohepatitis improve after rapid weight loss, but improvement also occurs after gradual weight reduction. It appears that in the future, weight loss, combined with PPRA-α or PPRA-γ agonist, will find a place in the treatment of NASH, but in the meantime more evidence is required.

POLYCYSTIC OVARY SYNDROME

Q: What features does the polycystic ovary syndrome share with the metabolic syndrome?
The polycystic ovary syndrome (PCOS) is a common disorder affecting 5% to 10% percent of women of reproductive age. Key features of PCOS are oligomenorrhea, clinical or laboratory evidence of hyperandrogenism, and the absence of other endocrinal disorders such as congenital adrenal hyperplasia, hyperprolactinemia, thyroid dysfunction, and androgen-secreting tumors.

Women who suffer from PCOS have a high risk of developing type 2 diabetes (about two- to threefold relative to weight-matched controls) and CHD events. This risk is approximately 50% higher compared with age- and BMI-matched women without PCOS. Assessment should include fasting glucose estimation with a follow-up glucose tolerance test in those who have a raised fasting glucose and are obese or have a family history of PCOS. There is no need for routine lipid estimation as these patients' absolute risk is rather low, despite the higher relative risk of CHD, and clinical management probably remains unchanged. Peripheral insulin resistance is manifested more intensely in overweight women. Obesity and PCOS have a more synergic effect in the presence of insulin resistance.

Even if the adipose tissue and skeletal muscle are resistant to insulin, the ovary and adrenals may retain their normal response to insulin (and insulin-like growth factor-I [IGF-I]). As a result of this normal stimulating effect, there is an increase in thecal and stromal production within the ovary, leading to abnormal follicular development and finally to ovarian dysfunction and menstrual irregularities. The increased androgen level and hyperinsulinemia are associated with decreased circulating sex hormone–binding globulin (SHBG) (a carrier of circulating androgen), resulting in an elevated level of androgen activity (hirsutism, acne, and alopecia) [1]. Some women who have a lean body mass may not exhibit frank manifestations of insulin resistance but features only of increased ovarian sensitivity to insulin.

Lipids and Hemostatic Factors

Women with PCOS manifest many lipid abnormalities that are common with metabolic syndrome, such increased triglycerides, decreased HDL cholesterol, mildly elevated LDL cholesterol, and increased small, dense LDL particles. There is increased hepatic lipase activity, an enzyme critical to the generation of small, dense LDL particles [48]. Pirwany et al [48] have shown that despite the atherogenic tendency of the lipid profile in overweight and obese women with PCOS, in terms of absolute CHD risk the modest differences in lipid levels, when considered in conjunction with other risk factors (young age, blood pressure often not raised), result in a low 10-year risk of CHD events [48]. Therefore, the majority of women with PCOS are not appropriate for primary prevention therapy for CHD.

Studies show that the levels of factor VIIc, fibrinogen, D-dimer, and von Willebrand factor are not different in women with PCOS [49]. However, another study found elevations in PAI-1 and tissue-type plasminogen activator (t-PA) in small cohorts of women with PCOS [48]. The level of t-PA in women with PCOS, like women without, seems to be related to the degree of obesity and varies inversely with insulin sensitivity [49]. There is further evidence that neither lipid abnormalities nor hemostatic disturbances (e.g., PAI-1, t-PA) correlated with total circulatory testosterone level [48,49].

Inflammation

Women with PCOS seem to have increased concentration of CRP [49], independent of BMI, and linked to greater insulin resistance. Other inflammatory markers such as white blood cell elevations and interleukin-18 have also been shown to be elevated in women with PCOS [50].

Endothelial Dysfunction

Most but not all studies report endothelial dysfunction in women with PCOS. Endothelial dysfunction even in young, normal weight women with PCOS may be linked to both their relative greater insulin resistance and low-grade inflammation.

Obesity

About half of women with PCOS have central obesity or a higher WC or waist/hip ratio [50]. They have an increased risk of the metabolic syndrome. Obese women have twice the risk as compared to age-matched women in the general population. One study also observed that women who had the metabolic syndrome had higher free testosterone, lower SHBG, and a higher level of more acanthosis nigricans. Despite these metabolic abnormalities, it remains far from clear as to how extensively these women should be screened. However, recently it was suggested that they should have triglycerides, HDL cholesterol, blood pressure, and fasting glucose measured. In addition, selected women should have an oral glucose tolerance test (OGTT) [50], especially those women who have another component of the metabolic syndrome, such as obesity (BMI >30), fasting glucose >5.6 mmol/L (100 mg/L), or a family history of the metabolic syndrome.

Atherosclerosis and Coronary Heart Disease
A number of studies have shown an increased risk of vascular risk in women with PCOS based on the surrogate end points, including carotid intima-media wall thickness (IMT), coronary artery calcification, and angiography [1]. Studies do not substantiate an increased risk of CHD in women with PCOS. In one study there was approximately a 50% higher CHD risk relative to controls with adjustment for age, BMI, smoking, parity, and menstrual status.

Q: What aspects of treatment are common to the polycystic ovary syndrome and the metabolic syndrome?
Presently, there is no evidence of a long-term effect of lifestyle and insulin-sensitizing drugs in PCOS. However, a lifestyle benefit cannot be denied. A reduction of 5% to 10% in body weight in women with PCOS is associated with improvement of ovarian function and some metabolic abnormalities, such as improved fertility and improved risk factor profile. In this context, lifestyle measures including physical activities should be the first line of approach in clinical management.

Metformin
Metformin has a modest effect on ovulation and reduces gestational diabetes if taken throughout pregnancy. There is reduction of obesity, fasting insulin, t-PA, LDL cholesterol, and CRP, and increased HDL cholesterol. Metformin therefore reduced the risk of diabetes and likely the vascular risk in PCOS, but the evidence to support the reduction of CVD is lacking. Metformin tends to reduce BMI by around 4%, and total and free androgens are reduced by 20% (relative to placebo) [51]. A combination of diet and metformin for 6 months reduced the metabolic syndrome prevalence in women with PCOS [52].

PPARγ

Recent publications suggest that thiazolidinediones (TZDs) improve insulin resistance independent of BMI, SHBG, luteinizing hormone (LH), androgen levels, and the IGF axis, with parallel evidence of improved menstrual cycle/ovulation [53]. It appears that TZDs may be more effective in insulin resistance and endothelial dysfunction than metformin in women with PCOS. The TZDs can also improve reproductive and metabolic derangements and improve menstrual cyclicity in women not satisfactorily responsive to metformin [52]. Thus, there appears to be favorable effects on metabolic factors and reproductive outcome with TZDs. They improve liver function tests (with reduced γ-GT and ALT). There is an increase in subcutaneous fat vs. metformin. The effects on lipids are less studied, and the safety of these drugs during pregnancy needs to be investigated.

Orlistat

Orlistat reduces the risk of type 2 diabetes in obese subjects, resulting in greater weight loss (5%) as compared to metformin, but there are equivalent effects in reducing testosterone, and it had no effect on insulin sensitivity and lipids [54].

SLEEP APNEA

Q: Is there evidence that sleep apnea is related to the metabolic syndrome and cardiovascular Disease?

Obstructive sleep apnea (OSA) is associated with increased CV morbidity and mortality. It is independently associated with the CV risk factors that comprise metabolic syndrome and its overall prevalence [55]. It also is independently associated with increased systolic and diastolic blood pressure, increased fasting insulin level, elevated triglycerides, low HDL cholesterol, and increased total cholesterol/HDL ratio, but not with fasting glucose [55]. It is likely that OSA either directly increases the risk factors associated with the metabolic syndrome, or OSA and the metabolic syndrome share a common risk factor other than obesity, such as a sedentary lifestyle [55]. One study found that OSA and the metabolic syndrome share a similar pathophysiologic milieu that would be expected to increase the risk of CVD [56]. It has been suggested that increased TNF-α, IL-6, high sensitive, CRP (hsCRP) are involved in the pathogenesis of systemic inflammation in OSA [57]. It has also been suggested that OSA is related to obesity, insulin resistance, and diabetes mellitus. One study has found that levels of adiponectin in the blood are decreased as the level of TNF-α, IL-6, hsCRP, and adhesion molecules, monocyte chemotactic protein-1 (MCP-1) were markedly and significantly elevated in patients with OSA as compared to controls. Another study found that sleep apnea in obese middle-aged men is associated with visceral obesity, inflammatory cytokines elevation, hyperleptinemia, and hyperinsulinemia [58]. It was suggested that progressive deterioration of sleep apnea may accelerate the worsening of visceral obesity and the metabolic syndrome by providing a stress stimulus and causing nocturnal elevation of hormones, such as cortisol and insulin, that promote visceral adiposity, metabolic abnormalities, and CV complications [58]. A study shows that OSA (and sleep deprivation, such as in shift work) may independently lead to the metabolic syndrome. The converse may also be true, in that metabolic abnormalities associated with the metabolic syndrome and insulin resistance may potentially exacerbate sleep disorders [59].

References

1. Byrne CD, Wild SH. The Metabolism Syndrome. New York: John Wiley & Sons, 2005.
2. Lakka H-M, Laaksonen DE, Lakha TA, et al. The metabolic syndrome and total and CVD mortality in middle-aged men. JAMA 2002;288:2709–2716.
3. Hunt KJ, Resendez WK, Haffner SM, et al. NCEP vs. WHO metabolic in relation to all-cause and CV mortality in the San Antonio Heart Study. Circulation 2004;110:1251–1257.
4. Grundy SM. Metabolic syndrome: connecting and reconciling CV and diabetes world. J Am Coll Cardiol 2006;47:1093–1100.
5. Li TY, Rana JS, Manson JE, et al. Obesity as compared with physical activity in predicting risk of CHD in women. Circulation 2006;113:499–506.
6. Lorenzo C, Okoloise M, Williams K, et al. The metabolic syndrome as predictor of type 2 diabetes: the San Antonio Heart Study. Diabetes Care 2003;26(11):3153-3159.
7. Malik S, Wong ND, Franklin SS, et al. Impact of the metabolic syndrome on mortality for CHD, CVD, and all causes in US. Circulation 2004;110:1245–1250.
8. Bonora E, Targher G, Formentini G, et al. The metabolic syndrome is an independent predictor of CVD in type 2 diabetes subjects. Prospective data. Diabet Med 2004;21:52.
9. Ninomiya JK, L'Italien G, Crighi MH, et al. Association of metabolic syndrome with history of myocardial infarction and stroke in the 3rd NHANES survey. Circulation 2004;109:42–46.
10. Palter MK, Meigs JB, Sullivan LM, et al. CRP, the metabolic syndrome and prediction of CV events in the Framingham Offspring Study. Circulation 2004;110:380–385.
11. Hu G, Qiao Q, Tuomilehto J, et al. Prevalence of the metabolic syndrome and its relation to all-cause and CVD mortality in non-diabetic European men and women. Arch Intern Med 2004;164:1066–1076.

12. Lakka HM, Lakka TA, Tuomilehto J, et al. Abdominal obesity is associated with increased risk of coronary events in men. Eur Heart J 2002;23:706.

13. Hsia J, Bitter V, Tripputi M, et al. Metabolic syndrome and coronary angiographic disease progression: the Women's Angiographic Vitamin and Estrogen Trial. Am Heart J 2003;146:439–445.

14. Ridker PM, Buring JE, Cook NR, et al. CRP, the metabolic syndrome, and risk of incident CV events: an 8-year follow-up of 14 719 initially healthy American women. Circulation 2003;107:391–397.

15. Alexander CM, Landsman PB, Teutsch SM, et al. NCEP-defined metabolic syndrome, diabetes and prevalence of CHD among NHANES III participants age 50 years and older. Diabetes 2003;52:1210–1214.

16. Guzder RN, Gatling W, Mulleo MA, et al. Impact of metabolic syndrome criteria on CVD risk in people with newly diagnosed type 2 diabetes. Diabetologia 2006;49:49–55.

17. Iribarren C, Go AS, Husson G, et al. Metabolic syndrome and early-onset CAD. Is the whole greater than its parts. J Am Coll Cardiol 2006;48(9):1800–1807.

18. Wilson P, D'Agostino R, Parise H, et al. Metabolic syndrome as a precursor of CVD and type 2 diabetes. Circulation 2005;112:3066–3072.

19. Gami AS, Witt BJ, Howard DE, et al. Metabolic syndrome and risk of incident CVD events and death. J Am Coll Cardiol 2007;49:403–414.

20. Ninomiya JK, L'Halien G, Crigui MH, et al. Association of the metabolic syndrome with history of myocardial infarction and stroke in the third NHANES survey. Circulation 2004;109:42–46.

21. Ferrannini E, Natali A, Bell P, et al. Insulin resistance and hypersecretion in obesity. J Clin Invest 1997;100:1166–1173.

22. Ford ES, Mukdad AH, Giles WH. Trends in waist circumference among US adults. Obes Res 2003;11:1223–1231.

23. Gordon T, Castelli WP, Hjortland MC, et al. HDL as a protective factor against CHD. The Framingham Study. Am J Med 1977;62:707–714.

24. Relationship between baseline risk factors and CHD and total mortality in the Multiple Risk Factor Intervention Trial. Prev Med 1986;15:254–273.

25. Assman G, Schulte H. Role of triglycerides in CVD: lessons from the Prospective Cardiovascular Munster Study. Am J Cardiol 1992;70:10H–13H.

26. Hopkins PN, Wu LL, Hunt SC, et al. Plasma triglycerides and type II hyperlipidemia are independently associated with premature familial CAD. J Am Coll Cardiol 2005;45:1003–1012.

27. Klein BE, Klein R, Lee KE. Components of metabolic syndrome and risk of CVD and diabetes in Beaver Dam. Diabetes Care 2002;25:1790–1794.

28. Yip J, Facchini FS, Reaven GM. Resistance to insulin-mediated glucose disposal as a predictor of CVD. J Clin Endocrinol Metab 1998;83:2773–2776.

29. Lamarche B, St. Pierre AC, Rue IL, et al. A prospective population-based study of low density lipoprotein particle size as a risk factor for ischemic heart disease in men. Can J Cardiol 2001;17:859–865.

30. Stampfer MJ, Krauss RM, Ma J, et al. A prospective study of triglyceride level, LDL particle size diameter, and risk of myocardial infarction. JAMA 1996;276:882–888.

31. Freedman DS, Otvus JD, Jeyarajah EJ, et al. Relation of lipoprotein subclasses as measured by proton nuclear magnetic resonance spectroscopy to CAD. Arterioscler Thromb Vasc Biol 1998;18:1046–1053.

32. Walldius G, Juugner I, Holme I, et al. High ApoB B, low apoB A-I, and improvement in the prediction of fatal myocardial infarction: a prospective study. Lancet 2001;358:2026–2033.

33. Havel RJ. Role of triglyceride-rich lipoprotein in progression of atherosclerosis. Circulation 1990;81:694–696.

34. Hodis HN, Mack WJ, Azeu SP, et al. Triglyceride- and cholesterol-rich lipoproteins have a different effect on mild/moderate and severe lesion progression as assessed by quantitative coronary angiography in a controlled trial of lovastatin. Circulation 1994;90:42–49.

35. Sacks FM, Alaupovic P, Moye LA, et al. VLDL, apoB, CIII, E, and risk of recurrent CV in the CARE trial. Circulation 2000;102:1886–1892.

36. Schaefer EJ, McNamaro JR, Shah PK, et al. Elevated RLPs-cholesterol and triglyceride levels in diabetic men and women in the Framingham Offspring Study. Diabetes Care 2002;25:989–994.

37. Neuschwander-Tetri BA. Nonalcoholic steatohepatitis and the metabolic syndrome. Am J Med Sci 2005;333:326–335.

38. Day CP. NASH: Where are we now and where are we going? Gut 2002;50:585–588.

39. Marchesini G, Brizi M, Morselli-Labate AM, et al. Association of NAFLD with insulin resistance. Am J Med 1999;107(5):450–455.

40. Neuschwander-Teri BA. Fatty liver and the metabolic syndrome. Curr Opin Gastroenterol 2007;23:193–198.

41. Leclercq IA. Antioxidant defense mechanism: new players in the pathogenesis of non-alcoholic steatohepatitis. Clin Sci (Lond) 2004;106(3):235–237.

42. Videla LA, Rodrigo R, Orellana M, et al. Oxidative stress-related parameters in liver of non-alcoholic fatty liver disease patients. Clin Sci (Lond) 2004;106(3):261–268.

43. Xu A, Wang Y, Keshaw H, et al. The fat-derived hormone adiponectin alleviates alcoholic and nonalcoholic fatty liver disease in mice. J Clin Invest 2003;112(1):91–100.

44. Shimomura I, Bashmakov Y, Horton JD, et al. Increased level of nuclear SREBP-1c associated with fatty livers in two mouse models of diabetes mellitus. J Biol Chem 1999;274(42):30028–30032.

45. Zhou G, Myers R, Li Y, et al. Role of AMP-activated protein kinase in mechanism of metformin action. J Clin Invest 2001;108(8):1167–1174.

46. Neuschwander-Teri BA, Brunt EM, Wehmeier KR, et al. Improved nonalcoholic steatohepatitis after 48 weeks of treatment with the PPAR-γ ligand rosiglitazone. Hepatology 2003;38(4):1008–1017.

47. Promrat K, Lutchman G, Uwaifo GI, et al. A pilot study of pioglitazone treatment for nonalcoholic steatohepatitis. Hepatology 2004;39(1):188–196.

48. Pirwany IR, Fleming R, Greer IA, et al. Lipids and lipoprotein subfraction in women with PCOS: relationship to metabolic and endocrine parameters. Clin Endocrinol (Oxf) 2001;54:447–453.

49. Kelly CJ, Lyall H, Petrie JR, et al. A specific elevation in tissue plasminogen activator antigen in women with PCOS. J Clin Endocrinol Metab 2002;87:3287–3290.

50. Escobar-Morreale HF, Botella-Carretero JI, Villuendal G, et al. Serum IL-18 concentrations are increased in the PCOS: relationship to insulin resistance and to obesity. J Clin Endocrinol Metab 2004;89:806–811.

51. Horborne L, Fleming R, Lyall H, et al. Descriptive reviews of the evidence for the use of metformin in PCOS. Lancet 2003;361:1894–1901.

52. Glueck CJ, Papanna R, Wang P, et al. Incidence and treatment of metabolic syndrome in newly referred women with confirmed PCOS. Metabolism 2003;52:908–915.

53. Belli SH, Graffigna MN, Oneto A, et al. Effect of rosiglitazone on insulin resistance, growth factors, and reproductive disturbances in women with PCOS. Fertil Steril 2004;81:624–629.

54. Jayagopal V, Kilpatrick ES, Holding S, et al. Orlistat beneficial as metformin in the treatment of PCOS. J Clin Endocrinol Metab 2004;90:729–733.

55. Coughlin SR, Mawdsley L, Mugarza JA. Obstruction sleep apnea is independently associated with an increased prevalence of metabolic syndrome. Eur Heart J 2004;25:735–741.

56. Gami AS, Somers VK. OSA and metabolic syndrome and CV outcome. Eur Heart J 2004;25:709–711.

57. Teramoto S, Yamamoto H, Yamaguchi Y, et al. OSA causes systemic inflammation and metabolic syndrome. Chest 2005;127:1074–1075.

58. Alexandros N, Vgoutzas, Dimitris A, et al. Sleep apnea and day time sleepiness and fatigue. J Clin Endocrinol Metab 200;85:1151–1158.

59. Wolk R, Somers VK. Sleep apnea and hypertension. Exp Physiol 2007;92:67–68.

60. Meigs JB, Wilson PW, Nathan DM et al. Prevalence and characteristics of the metabolic syndrome in the San Antonio and Framingham Offspring Studies. Diabetes 2003;52:2160–2167.

Chapter 6
Clinical Management of the Metabolic Syndrome

RISK ASSESSMENT

Q: What are the implications and methods for cardiovascular risk assessment for the metabolic syndrome?

Even though there is considerable doubt regarding the value of the metabolic syndrome as a cardiovascular disease (CVD) risk marker, it is important to estimate the 10-year risk for CVD (or coronary heart disease [CHD]) in individuals with the metabolic syndrome because the intensity of management of risk factors in the metabolic syndrome depends on the global risk of CVD. It is an erroneous concept that the presence of the metabolic syndrome indicates high risk, similar to that of established CHD or type 2 diabetes. The absolute risk in the metabolic syndrome is variable, and some individuals are at only moderate or moderately high risk for CVD. In the absence of diabetes, individuals with the metabolic syndrome are not necessarily at a high 10-year risk. Besides, risk factors of the metabolic syndrome are not graded for severity as are the risk factor equations considered in the Framingham scoring. It also does not include all the risk factors that are required in standard risk prediction algorithms. Therefore, the metabolic syndrome per se is not a suitable tool to estimate the 10-year risk for CHD. However, studies have shown that middle-aged people with the metabolic syndrome are at an increased absolute risk for CVD in the near future (e.g., 10-year risk) [1]. Long-term (lifetime) risk for CVD is increased sometimes even in those individuals who do not have a high 10-year risk. This situation arises in young adults who suffer from the metabolic syndrome. An important provoking factor that increases the lifetime risk for CVD is increased susceptibility for developing premature type 2 diabetes. In this group of patients, therapeutic lifestyle modification is the first-line therapy, but if the 10-year risk is high, drug therapy is indicated to mitigate CVD risk factors.

Several diagnostic engines are available for estimation of the 10-year risk for CVD (or CHD). These methods include major risk factors for CVD, such as cigarette smoking, hypertension, total cholesterol, high-density lipoprotein (HDL) cholesterol, age, gender, and sometimes other risk factors such as diabetes. Diabetes however should be considered for secondary prevention only. Risk assessment algorithms, such as those of the Framingham point scoring system (www.nhlbi.nih.gov/guidelines/cholesterol/risk-tbl.htm) in the United States or the Prospective Cardiovascular Munster (PROCAM) study in Germany, or the European risk prediction system called SCORE (Systemic Coronary Risk Evaluation [www.escardio.org]), and Joint British Societies CVD risk assessment charts in the United Kingdom (www.hyp.ac.uk/bhs/) are the most commonly and widely available for estimating multifactorial absolute risk in the clinical practice.

According to the Adult Treatment Panel (ATP-III) guidelines, risk assessment for CHD should be carried out by using the Framingham risk scoring [2], which categorizes patients into three risk categories, based on the 10-year risk for CHD: high risk (>20%), moderately high risk (10% to 20%), or low to moderate risk (<10%). The Framingham scoring takes into account age, gender, total cholesterol, smoking, HDL cholesterol, and systolic blood pressure. Some investigators from the Framingham Heart Study suggested that adding abdominal obesity, triglycerides, and fasting glucose to these parameters provides little or no increase in the power of prediction [3]. However, these parameters will be important in long-term management. Also, the CHD predictive power will improve by adding apolipoprotein B (ApoB), small low-density lipoprotein (LDL) particles, C-reactive protein (CRP), fibrinogen, and insulin level to these risk equations. Even risk algorithms based on established risk factors have a limited predictive power. Noninvasive imaging is an alternative promising technique [4]. The British Joint Societies' has a prediction chart that estimates CVD risk. Roughly, 20% CHD risk equals 15% CVD risk.

The Quebec Cardiovascular Study suggested that the simultaneous measurement and interpretation of waist circumference and fasting triglyceridemia could be used as inexpensive screening tools to identify men characterized by the atherogenic metabolic triad (hyperinsulinemia, elevated ApoB, and small, dense LDL) and a high risk of CHD [5]. The PROCAM risk algorithm also includes triglycerides and a family history of premature CHD [6]. The ATP-III guideline does not recommend using these measures routinely, but they should be considered as optional. If any of them is abnormal, the physician has the option to increase the risk accordingly.

The incidence of CVD among the Asian population is much less than in whites [7], and the Framingham risk scoring perhaps overestimates the risk of CHD in Asians. This is indicative of the fact that data based on the study of mainly white people are not exactly applicable to Asians. The value of adding risk factors such as abdominal obesity, Apo-B, small LDL cholesterol, CRP, and insulin and glucose levels to the current list used for defining the metabolic syndrome has not been adequately studied to prove if it will enhance prediction of CVD, whereas CRP appears to do so [3]. Diabetics who also have concurrently other metabolic syndrome factors are at high risk for future CVD.

GOALS FOR CLINICAL MANAGEMENT

Q: What are the goals of clinical management of the metabolic syndrome?
The primary goal of clinical management of patients with the metabolic syndrome is to reduce the risk of clinical atherosclerotic disease (Table 6.1). Emphasis should be placed on instigating lifestyle changes in the underlying risk factors, such as obesity, physical inactivity, and atherogenic diet. Lifestyle changes, if appropriately instituted, will reduce all the metabolic factors. General awareness of CVD risk among women is associated with preventive action. Educational interventions need to be targeted at racial/ethnic minority women. It is unknown whether treating insulin resistance itself would be of value in preventing CVD in all, or a subset, of the metabolic syndrome patients [7].

The ATP-III recommended that obesity be the primary target of intervention for the metabolic syndrome and that drug therapy should be used if necessary. First-line therapy is directed at the major risk factors such as elevated LDL cholesterol, hypertension, and diabetes. The only drugs approved for treatment are those that target the individual risk factors; lipid lowering drugs, antihypertensives, hypoglycemics, antiplatelets, and weight loss agents. For the use of these drugs the clinician should follow current guidelines from the National Cholesterol Education Program (NCEP 6th Joint program), the Joint National Committe (JNC's) seventh report, American Diabetes Association (ADA), American Heart Association (AHA)/American College of Cardiology (ACC), and the National Heart, Lung, and Blood Institute (NHLBI).

Candidate drugs for treatment of the metabolic syndrome as a whole and to reduce risk of CVD or diabetes are weight-reducing drugs, peroxisome proliferation–activated receptor-α (PPARα) agonists (fibrates), PPARγ agonists (thiazolidinediones [TZDs]), and dual

TABLE 6.1. National Cholesterol Education Program (NCEP) guidelines for the treatment of hyperlipidemia

Goals of therapy (Target LDL-C levels)	Therapeutic recommendations
High-risk[a] <100 mg/dL (2.6 mmol/L), but for very high risk it is <70 mg/dL (1.8 mmol/L) even if baseline LDL cholesterol <100 mg/dL	Lifestyle therapies plus LDL cholesterol therapy; if baseline LDL cholesterol ≥100 mg/dL (2.6 mmol/L), initiate/intensify LDL therapy; if baseline LDL cholesterol <100 mg/dL (2.6 mmol/L), initiate LDL therapy on clinical judgment; for elevated triglycerides or low HDL cholesterol, a fibrate or nicotinic acid with an LDL therapy
Moderately high-risk[b] <130 mg/dL (3.4 mmol/L) but <100 mg/dL (2.6 mmol/L) is optional	If baseline LDL cholesterol ≥130 mg/dL (3.4 mmol/L), LDL therapy after lifestyle therapies; if baseline LDL cholesterol is 100 (2.6 mmol/L) to 129 mg/dL (3.39 mmol/L), consider LDL therapy if patient's risk is in upper range
Moderate risk[c], <130 mg/dL (3.4 mmol/L)	If LDL cholesterol >160 mg/dL (4.2 mmol/L), LDL therapy after lifestyle therapies
Lower-risk[d], <160 mg/dL (4.2 mmol/L)	LDL therapy if LDL ≥190 mg/dL (4.9 mmol/L), but optional if 160 mg/dL (4.2 mmol/L) to 189 mg/dL (4.89 mmol/L) after dietary therapy

[a]CHD or CHD equivalent or 10-year risk for >20%.
[b]2+ risk factors (10-year risk 10% to 20%).
[c]2+ major risk factors (10-year risk <10%).
[d]0 to 1 risk factor (10-year risk<10%).
LDL therapy, lipid-lowering therapy.
Source: NCEP 3rd report [53].

PPAR agonist. The PPARα and PPARγ agonists are already indicated in the metabolic syndrome. Presently, there are efforts going on to find a suitable combined PPARα and PPARγ agonist. Fibrates reduce the risk of CVD through treatment of atherogenic dyslipidemia, possibly because of their antiinflammatory properties. In the analysis of the Scandinavian Simvastatin Survival Study (4S), simvastatin reduced CVD events to the same extent in nondiabetic patients with or without the metabolic syndrome [8]. Two weight-loss drugs, sibutramine and orlistat, are already approved by the Food and Drug Administration (FDA). These drugs improve all the metabolic risk factors but produce only a moderate weight loss.

Although weight loss and exercise are the main component of the treatment of the metabolic syndrome, they are also equally important for all components of the metabolic syndrome when they occur in isolation. Rimonabant causes a 5% to 10% weight loss for up to 2 years, and might have a systemic action that independently reduces the risk factors for the metabolic syndrome. The TZDs reduce insulin resistance and modestly improve various metabolic risk factors. Cholesteryl ester-transfer protein (CETP) inhibitors and torcetrapid, which raises HDL when used alone or in combination with a statin, were expected to prove useful to treat the dyslipidemia of the metabolic syndrome where lifestyle changes fail and CV risk is high. But torcetrapid has been withdrawn due to increased mortality. Research, however, is ongoing to find an alternative drug in this group.

Another important goal in the treatment of the metabolic syndrome is to prevent type 2 diabetes mellitus. If patients already suffer from it, management should be intensified to reduce their higher risk for CVD. The indications for drug therapy are elevated LDL cholesterol, hypertension, and elevated glucose. Smoking cessation among cigarette smokers should be reinforced. Important strategies for the treatment can be summarized as (1) lifestyle; (2) metformin; (3) glitazones/TZDs (cause ↓ fatty acids, ↓ insulin resistance, ↑ HDL cholesterol, balancing against possible weight gain); and (4) rimonabant (produces ↓ waist circumference [WC], ↓ triglycerides, ↑ HDL cholesterol), antihypertensives (i.e. calcium channel blockers) and angiotensin-converting enzyme inhibitors [ACE-Is]).

MANAGEMENT OF UNDERLYING RISK FACTORS

Atherogenic and Diabetogenic Diet

Q: What modifications need to be implemented to manage atherogenic and diabetogenic diets?
Dietary recommendations are a key element in the management of CVD. There is substantial evidence that certain dietary patterns can affect CVD by modifying risk factors such as obesity, dyslipidemia, and hypertension, as well as factors involved in systemic inflammation, insulin sensitivity, oxidative stress, endothelial function, thrombosis, and cardiac rhythm [10].

Presently, the typical American diet is estimated to derive 49% of its calories from carbohydrates, 34% from fat, and 12% to 16% from protein [10].

Weight Management

For weight management, intake of a low-calorie, low-fat diet is recommended. The principle behind a low-fat diet for weight management is based on fat's greater energy value (9 kcal/g [38 kJ]) and less for carbohydrate and protein (4 kcal/g [17 kJ]). A carbohydrate-modified diet may be a low-carbohydrate diet or a low-glycemic-index diet. A low-carbohydrate diet may be one alternative for weight reduction. The Atkins diet begins with an initial weight-loss induction phase in which carbohydrate intake is restricted to 20 g (as low as 5% of total calories) per day for at least 2 weeks. This is in sharp contrast to the ATP-III recommendation, which allocated 50% to 60% of total calories to carbohydrates. Subsequently, carbohydrate consumption is gradually increased but still remains below a critical level for continued weight loss or maintenance. The contents of various low-carbohydrate diets are as follows [10]:

- The Atkins diet contains carbohydrate (CHO) 5%, fat 68% (saturated fat 26%), and protein 27%.
- The Stillman diet contains CHO 3%, fat 33% (saturated fat 13%), and protein 64%.
- The Protein Power diet contains CHO 16%, fat 54% (saturated fat 18%), and protein 26%.
- The Zone diet contains CHO 36%, fat 29% (saturated fat 9%), and protein 34%.

The ATP-III recommendations for diet composition for patients with the metabolic syndrome are consistent with general dietary recommendations [11]. There is, however a general paucity of evidence of a direct link between diet and the development of the metabolic syndrome. The effects of diet on CHD is mediated through various pathways, the most important presently is through the inflammatory process. It has been suggested that inflammation strictly correlates with endothelial dysfunction and insulin resistance. The n-3 fatty acids may inhibit the synthesis of proinflammatory cytokines (e.g., tumor necrosis factor-α [TNF-α], interleukin-6 [IL-6], IL-2). Four dietary strategies are recommended for the prevention of CHD: (1) Increase n-3 from plant and fish sources. (2) Substitute nonhydrogenated unsaturated fats for saturated and *trans* fats. (3) Consume a diet high in fruits, vegetables, nuts, and whole grains, and low in refined grains.

(4) Reduce salt (<3 g/d) and calorie intake. Several studies have shown an inverse association between the n-3 polyunsaturated fatty acids (PUFAs), α-linolenic acid, eicosapentaenoic acid (EPA), and docosahexaenoic acid (DHA), and serum levels of inflammatory markers in healthy subjects and those with stable coronary artery disease (CAD) [11]. The n-3 PUFA-rich diets and dietary fiber also appear to be inversely associated with CRP level. Nut and seed consumption has also been suggested to be inversely correlated with CRP, IL-6, and fibrinogen levels, especially in whites [10]. Very low fat diets are based on variations of vegetarian diets but contain fat <15% (vs. ATP-III 25% to 35%) of total calories.

Fats

Fats are either saturated or unsaturated, and the latter are either mono- (MUFAs) or polyunsaturated fatty acids (PUFAs). The polyunsaturates are of linoleic acid (n-6) and α-linolenic acid (n-3) subtypes. The type of fat in the diet can affect serum lipids to a greater extent than the absolute amount of fat. *Trans* fatty acids, derived from industrial hydrogenation of PUFAs, raise LDL and lipoprotein (a) levels and decrease HDL levels. Saturated fatty acids increase LDL and HDL levels. Dietary cholesterol can increase total cholesterol and LDL levels to a lesser extent than do saturated fatty acids. The MUFAs and PUFAs affect the lipid profile favorably by lowering LDL and raising HDL levels.

It is advisable to avoid excessive fat intake, reduce saturated fatty acids, and replace monosaturated fatty acids and some polyunsaturated fatty acids with a *cis* configuration. A low-fat diet (≤30% of total calories) is considered by clinicians to be healthy for both primary and secondary prevention of CVD, but prescribing a low-fat diet may give the patient a misleading message that an unrestricted carbohydrate intake is allowed, when in fact it is unsuitable as it reduces HDL cholesterol and increases triglycerides, exacerbating the metabolic manifestations of the metabolic syndrome. Higher intake of *trans* fats or, to a lesser extent, saturated fats have been shown to be associated with increased CHD risk among 80,082 women in the Nurses' Health Study cohort, where higher intake of polysaturated (nonhydrogenated) and monosaturated fats was associated with decreased risk [13]. A positive correlation between saturated fats and plasma biomarkers of inflammation has been demonstrated.

The ATP-III [4] recommends that patients' cholesterol intake be managed; the dietary total fat should be 25% to 35% of calories. If it exceeds 35%, then it is difficult to maintain the low intake of saturated fat, which is required to maintain a low LDL cholesterol.

On the other hand, if dietary fat content falls below 25%, then triglycerides can rise and HDL cholesterol levels can decline. Hence, a very low fat diet may exacerbate atherogenic dyslipidemia. To avoid worsening atherogenic dyslipidemia, some investigators advocate a fat intake of 30% to 35%, while others advise 25% to 30% due to possible weight gain caused by long-term intake of higher fat [11]. A few studies have suggested there are CV benefits from very low fat diets, but the inclusion of lifestyle changes, such as aerobic exercise and stress management, confused the issue in these studies.

Dietary Fat and Insulin Sensitivity
A diet that is high in fat, though energy-rich, does not provide satiety. It is not certain if total dietary fat has any appreciable effect on insulin resistance and on other metabolic features of the metabolic syndrome, but the benefits of weight loss on insulin sensitivity thus achieved remain undisputed. In the Kuopio, Aarhus, Naples, Wollongong, Uppsala (KANWU) study, a change of the proportions of dietary fatty acids, decreasing saturated fatty acids and increasing monosaturated fatty acid, improved insulin sensitivity but had no effect on insulin secretion. A beneficial impact of fat quality (substituting MUFAs for saturated) is not seen in individuals with a high fat intake (>37 Energy%) [13]. It is more widely accepted that saturated fats impair insulin action while n-3 unsaturated fatty acids improve it. Monosaturated and n-6 polyunsaturated fatty acids have a less significant effect on insulin sensitivity. A normal-fat diet with replacement of saturated by unsaturated fatty acids has the following effects: (1) reduction of weight; (2) improvement in insulin sensitivity; (3) improvement in the lipid profile (i.e., reduction in very low density lipoprotein [VLDL] triglycerides, and reduction in LDL cholesterol; and (4) reduction in blood pressure [13].

Polyunsaturated fatty acids of both the n-6 and n-3 classes are inversely related to the risk of CHD. Linoleic acid is the main fatty acid in the n-6 group, and is principally found in vegetable oils. α-Linolenic acid is the precursor of the n-3 group (EPA and DHA), and the main sources are certain vegetable oils: soybean, safflower, linseed oils, canola, flaxseed, and walnut oil; nuts; and vegetables of the cabbage family, lettuce, cabbage, and other green vegetables. A diet rich in α-linolenic acid (Lyon Diet Heart Study) in high-risk individuals reduces coronary mortality and all-cause mortality [14]. The n-3 class EPA and DHA are mainly obtained from fish (fatty fish [especially salmon and anchovy], sardines, herring, mackerel, lake trout; and some vegetable oils such as soybean). It has been suggested that a lower intake of n-6 PUFA may be related to the presence of metabolic abnormalities in South Asians, but none of the dietary contents of the South Asian diet was associated with a higher CHD risk in the Southall study [15].

In the Western diet, the principal n-6 PUFA is linoleic acid, which is found in safflower, sunflower, and corn oils. Studies show that supplementation of the diet with n-3 PUFA had no effect on insulin action in individuals on either a moderate or high n-6 PUFA diet. In postprandial state triglyceride concentrations were reduced by a greater amount in people consuming a high n-6 background diet subsequent to fish oil supplementation rich in n-3 PUFA [16]. Dietary fat should predominantly be monosaturated fats (e.g., oleic acid) and with modest intake of n-6 polyunsaturated fatty acids and some n-3 fatty acids. Monosaturates are derived from vegetable sources (e.g., olive oil). They can assist in the reduction of saturated fat, and there is tentative evidence that a modest intake of monosaturated fatty acids can reduce the risk of macrovascular disease. Increments in insulin sensitivity may become directly related to the loss of intramyocellular or omental fat rather than body weight per se.

Fish

Besides containing protein and other nutrients (e.g., vitamins and selenium), fish (either fin-fish or shellfish, and especially salmon, sardines, and herring) contain omega-3 fatty acid, which may reduce the risk of developing CHD and other medical problems. The n-3 fatty acids can help lower blood pressure, heart rate, and other CV risk factors. Eating fish reduces the risk of death from heart disease and lowers the risk of stroke, depression, and mental decline with age. For pregnant and lactating mothers and women of childbearing age, fish intake supplies DHA, which is beneficial for the developing brain of infants. However, fish may contain mercury, which may have mysterious effects on the developing nervous system in infants. Therefore, women who are pregnant or may become pregnant, lactating mothers, and very young children should avoid shark, swordfish, king mackerel, and golden bass. The FDA Web site can provide information on the mercury content of some fish; go to www.cfsan.fda.gov/~dms/admehg3.html.

Carbohydrates

The carbohydrate type affects the CHD risk. Refined carbohydrates are highly processed, resulting in the removal of fiber, vitamins, minerals, phytonutrients, and essential fatty acids. A high intake of refined starches and sugar causes rapid swings in blood sugar and insulin level, which may increase hunger and may elevate the free fatty acid (FFA) level. A very high dietary content of carbohydrates can aggravate the dyslipidemia of the metabolic syndrome. The long-term effects of a low-carbohydrate diet have not been studied adequately in patients with the metabolic syndrome, although the short-term effects show benefits, such as lower triglyceride level, raised HDL cholesterol, and reduced body weight. An alternative to lower consumption of all carbohydrates is to replace high glycemic index foods with less refined, lower glycemic index foods that contain more fiber. Low glycemic index food produces lower levels of postprandial glucose and lower levels of insulin. Current fiber intake is below the recommended levels, and limiting the grain intake will make this worse. A low glycemic index diet has been suggested as a treatment for obesity. A firm correlation of carbohydrate-modified diets and low-carbohydrate diets with glycemic load with CAD has not yet been established.

Sterols/Stenols
Dietary plant sterols and their saturated counterpart stenols have been observed to lower the cholesterol level. Plant sterols or stenols that have been esterified to increase their lipid solubility can be incorporated into food, and will reduce the absorption of cholesterol from the gut and will lower the blood cholesterol. Two grams of plant stenol or sterol added to an average portion of margarine reduces LDL cholesterol by an average of 0.54 mmol/L in middle-aged individuals. A reduction of about 0.5 mmol/L of LDL cholesterol will reduce the risk of CHD by approximately 25% over 2 years. There is good evidence now that dietary modification using a diet high in plant sterol (e.g., Benacana, Proactive), soy protein, and viscous fibers and almond lower inflammatory markers such as CRP, IL-6, white blood cell count, and fibrinogen [17].

Soya
In a review of soy protein trials by the America Heart Association (AHA) Nutrition Committee, ingestion of soy protein (25 to 135 g/d) containing isoflavones (40 to 318 mg/d) was associated with a 3% weighted average reduction in LDL and non-HDL cholesterol levels; the effects on HDL and triglyceride levels were small (+1.5% and –5%, respectively) and not significant in most studies. In 19 studies that tested the effect of isoflavones on lipids, the weighted average reduction in LDL was 0%. Thus, current evidence favors soy protein, not soy isoflavones, as the important factor in LDL lowering [11].

Dietary Fiber and the Glycemic Index

Dietary fiber may play a role in circulating insulin levels. Dietary fiber reduces insulin secretion by slowing the rate of nutrient absorption following a meal. Insulin sensitivity increases and weight decreases on high-fiber diets. Also, fiber protects against hypertension, hyperlipidemia, and CVD. A high-fiber intake has a favorable effect on total cholesterol and LDL level. Soluble fiber is well known to reduce cholesterol. In addition, oat products seem to decrease the concentration of small, dense LDL particles.

In the diabetic individual, the glycemic control also may be affected unfavorably and plasminogen activator inhibitor-1 (PAI-1) is raised on a high carbohydrate diet, indicating enhanced thrombogenic tendency. Many of these problems can be avoided by if the carbohydrate is rich in dietary fiber, especially the soluble form (e.g., oat, barley, seeds [especially phylum], rye, fruits, vegetables, wheat). Many of the carbohydrate containing-foods have a low glycemic index (GI).

The glycemic index refers to the increase in blood glucose that occurs after consuming a fixed amount (usually 50 g) of available carbohydrates from a test food relative to the increase in blood glucose that occurs after consuming the same amount of available carbohydrates from either glucose or white bread [18]. Foods containing a low GI (e.g., cereals, rice, and pasta) have a low postprandial rise, associated with slow digestion and absorption. The GI of some foods is as follows: Kellogg's All Bran cereal, 51; Kellogg's Corn Flakes cereal, 84; oatmeal, 49; Basmati rice, 58; noodles (instant), 46; spaghetti, 43; a bagel, 72; yogurt (low-fat), 33; banana, 55; orange, 44; broccoli, 10; potato (baked), 93; and lentils, 30. Low-GI diets are the following [10]:

- Montana diet: Up to 30% to 40% CHO, but only those with a GI <35 are allowed during weight-losing phase; there is more emphasis on GI in subsequent phases.
- Sugar Busters diet: 52% CHO (emphasis on CHO with low GI), fat 21% (saturated fat 4%), protein 27%.
- South Beach diet: Extreme CHO restriction for 2 weeks, followed by reintroduction of CHO with low GI; also encourages intake of MUFAs, PUFAs, fiber, and lean protein.

Starchy food is readily digested and absorbed as glucose, giving rise to a marked rapid postprandial glycemia. Acute hyperglycemia impairs endothelial-dependent vasodilatation and reduces NO availability. Coronary heart disease may be more related to post-load glucose hyperglycemia than to fasting hyperglycemia. High-GI foods can increase triglycerides and cause other metabolic abnormalities. Conversely, low-GI foods, such as a diet high in fiber, are associated with a lower insulin response. It is interesting that most if not all low-GI foods are also high in fiber. Food rich in soluble fiber and with a high amylase-to-amylopectin content ratio (e.g., parboiled rice, legumes) have a low GI. Most refined produce and potatoes have a high GI, whereas most fruits, legumes, and nonstarchy vegetables have a low GI [18].

The glycemic load is the product of GI and the carbohydrate content of one serving of that food. It is more reasonable measure because it takes into account both the quantity and the quality of the carbohydrate taken. For example, watermelon has a GI of 72, which is high, but it contains only 5% of carbohydrate (one portion of watermelon), and its calculated glycemic load is 4, which is low. Low-energy-density food is another alternative choice for weight reduction. The energy density of a diet can be defined as the calories derived from a given weight of food. The energy density of a particular food directly correlates with its fat content and inversely correlates with its water content [18]. Parboiled rice and certain type of pasta have a low GI but are not especially high in fiber [19]. Reducing the GI in the diet without altering the energy balance, the proportion of carbohydrate and fat or the amount of dietary fat can favorably affect several components of the metabolic syndrome including PAI-1 [19].

Nuts

An inverse association between nuts consumption and CHD risk has been consistently found. The beneficial effects are found in walnuts, cashews, and Brazil nuts. Nuts are rich in mono- and polyunsaturated fatty acids, which makes them a palatable choice for healthy fats. Monosaturated fats may contribute to a decreased CHD risk [20] by (1) amelioration of the lipid profile, and (2) reduction of soluble inflammatory adhesion molecules in patients with hypercholesterolemia. In addition, the relatively high arginine content of nuts has been suggested as one of the potential mechanisms for the cardioprotective effect, because consumption of arginine-rich food is associated with lower CRP levels. There appears to be an inverse correlation between nut and seed consumption and body mass index (BMI). Weight loss may be explained due to incomplete digestion of nuts and seeds and subsequent enhancement of satiety. There is some indication that individuals on a nut-rich diet excrete more fat in their stools. Also, almonds decrease the LDL/HDL ratio.

A diet high in fruits, vegetables, nuts, and whole grains, and low in refined grains, is recommended. An inverse association between fruit and vegetable consumption and CVD has been reported. A low intake of fruits, berries, and vegetables is associated with excess mortality in men [21]. The antioxidant component of fruits and vegetables, including vitamins and flavonoids, contributes to their antiinflammatory effect. Dietary fiber intake is inversely associated with serum CRP level [22]. Vegetables, legumes, intact fruits, and whole-grain cereals are preferred sources of carbohydrates and a low GI when carbohydrate intake is at the low end of this range. The Mediterranean style of diet is suitable for individuals with the metabolic syndrome. A diet containing high carbohydrates, high fiber, and low fat, supplemented by exercise to induce weight loss, had a favorable effect on insulin sensitivity, but only if enforced vigorously [23]. High-fiber, high-carbohydrate diets comprised of food with low caloric density can be used for effective weight reduction and to ameliorate insulin resistance. Although some data suggest that low-GI foods are more beneficial in this respect, these effects may have more to do with increments in dietary fiber than with differences in available carbohydrates. Studies show that the short-term benefits (e.g., weight loss, improved insulin sensitivity) obtained by a high-fat, low-carbohydrate diet (e.g., Atkins) and a high-protein diet (e.g., Zone diet, South Beach diet) are lost after 1 year [24].

Various Diets

A study reported the findings of a randomized trial in which the Mediterranean diet, which entails an increased intake of whole grains, fruits, vegetables, nuts, and olive oil, led to lower levels of high-sensitivity (hs)CRP (hsCRP), IL-6, IL-7, and IL-8, reduced insulin resistance, and improved endothelial function [25]. In the Gruppo Italiano per lo Studio della Sopravvivenza nell'Infarto Miocardio (GISSI) Prevenzione trial, patients randomized to receive n-3 fatty acid supplementation (1 g/d) had a significant 10% to 15% reduction in the combined primary end points of death and fatal/nonfatal stroke [9]. In the Lyon Diet Heart Study, patients on a Mediterranean diet rich in α-linolenic acid instead of a Western diet had a reduction in death from CV causes: nonfatal acute myocardial infarction by 73%, CV mortality by 76%, and all-cause mortality by 70% [14]. A Mediterranean diet generally entails an abundance of plant food (vegetables, legumes, fruits, nuts, and whole-grain cereals), with olive oil as the main source of fat, and a moderately high intake of fish, a relatively low intake of meat and poultry, and a moderate consumption of wine.

In the Diet and Reinfarction Trial (DART), men recovering from a myocardial infarction who were randomized to receive dietary advice recommending increased fatty fish consumption had a 29% reduction in all-cause mortality at the 2-year follow-up [26]. The Dietary Approaches to Stop Hypertension (DASH) diet can likely reduce most of the metabolic risks in both men and women, but the related mechanism needs further study [27]. The DASH diet reduced the prevalence of the metabolic syndrome by one third. The DASH eating plan includes a diet rich in fruits, vegetables, and low fat dairy products, with reduced content of cholesterol and saturated and total fat. It limits sodium to 3 g/d, and is rich in potassium and calcium.

Alcohol

Q: What is the role of alcohol in the prevention of coronary heart disease and the metabolic syndrome?
There is a well-established relationship between alcohol intake and CHD risk. A higher risk is associated both with high consumption and with teetotalism. The maximum weekly recommended intake in the United Kingdom is 21 units (a maximum of three units per day) for men and 14 units (a maximum of two units per day) for women. This is better taken on regular basis. The United States guidelines recommend a maximum of two drinks for men (1 oz or 30 mL ethanol, e.g., 24 oz of beer, 10 oz of wine, or 3 oz of 80 proof whisky per day) and no more than one drink per day for women. A unit of alcohol in the U.K. is 8 g of ethanol, in the U.S. is 12 to 14 g, in Austria is 6.3 g, and in Japan is 19.75 g. Eight grams of alcohol is equivalent to 10 mL of pure alcohol. A drink in U.S. is 12 oz of beer, 5 oz of wine, or 1.5 oz of 80-proof liquor. In the U.K. one unit is equal to 30 mL (1 fluid oz) of spirits (whisky, Vodka, brandy), 300 mL of normal beer, or one glass (120 mL or 4 oz) of wine. One gram of alcohol provides 7 kcal/g of energy. Moderate consumption of alcohol has beneficial effects on HDL and fibrinogen level and on platelet aggregation. Alcohol increases the HDL cholesterol level, which accounts for 50% of its cardioprotective effect. It also reduces the levels of inflammation. There is no evidence of any difference in CV benefit of any one source of alcohol compared with another [28]. However, some studies advocate that wine is more beneficial.

Two related components of drinking pattern are binge drinking and frequency of drinking. The pattern of alcohol use also has an effect on CV risk; binge drinking is associated with a higher risk of sudden death and stroke. Binge drinking is defined as consumption of three or more drinks within 1 to 2 hours [29]. Recent studies show that more frequent drinking, especially consumption several days a week or even daily, is associated with more favorable outcomes than only occasional or weekly [30]. Alcohol intake at least of 3 to 4 days a week is associated with a lower risk of myocardial infarction among men and women. This link is attributable to the relationship of alcohol with HDL cholesterol, fibrinogen, and hemoglobin A_{1c} (HbA$_{1c}$), which is now widely accepted [30]. Intake of more than three units of alcohol a day is associated with increased risk of hemorrhagic stroke, (and to a lesser extent ischemic stroke), a rise in both diastolic and systolic blood pressure, an increased risk of cardiac arrhythmias, cardiomyopathy, and sudden death.

Alcohol has different effects on the various components of the metabolic syndrome because it increases HDL cholesterol, triglycerides, and blood pressure. A study showed that alcohol had a positive association with the prevalence of the metabolic syndrome [31]. A cross-sectional population-based study of 60-year-old men and women in Sweden ($n = 4232$) showed that moderate wine drinkers generally had a healthier lifestyle than either nondrinkers or spirit drinkers [32]. In women, the metabolic syndrome was significantly more common in nondrinkers (20%, $p < .05$) and less common among wine drinkers (8%, $p < .01$), compared with a group with low alcohol intake.

Physical Activity

Q: What is the definition of physical activity?
Regular exercise increases type 1 (aerobic, red) muscle fibers with augmented insulin sensitivity by utilizing FFAs, whereas type 2 (anaerobic, white) fibers predominate in sedentary individuals, contributing to insulin resistance. Because physical inactivity is related to the development of the metabolic syndrome, a program of regular physical activity should be initiated. Physical activity is associated with successful weight reduction and weight maintenance, and it improves insulin sensitivity, increases lean body mass, and favorably affects many of the metabolic abnormalities associated with obesity and the metabolic syndrome. Those who have a higher lean body mass are less likely to develop insulin resistance, as a higher lean body mass is associated with greater glucose disposal.

The intensity of exercise represents the total amount of energy expended in physical activity. It can be defined in absolute or in relative terms. Absolute intensity represents the rate of energy expenditure during exercise and is expressed in metabolic equivalents (METs). One MET is equivalent to energy consumed during resting such as watching TV and is equal to 1 kcal/kg of body weight per hour. Daily activities such as housework or gardening (2 to 5 METs), walking at a pace of 3 to 4 mph (3 to 4 METs), and jogging (8 to 10 METs) consume more calories. Increased physical activity is necessary for maintenance of weight loss, but many individuals find it difficult to maintain a regular long-term exercise program.

Q: What are the benefits of physical activity in individuals with the metabolic syndrome?

Regular physical activity prevents the development of diabetes and CVD, and reduces symptoms in patients with well-established CVD. It also reduces the risk of chronic disease such as type 2 diabetes, obesity, osteoporosis, depression, and cancer of the breast and colon. Studies have found that obese or overweight individuals who are physically active (e.g., participate in at least 30 minutes of moderate-intensity physical activity on most days) or who have moderate to high levels of cardiorespiratory fitness have a much lower death rate from CVD and all-cause mortality than do individuals who are sedentary and unfit. Increasing physical activity benefits the metabolic risk factors, and it reduces the overall CVD risk. Recent guidelines for physical activity recommend regular, practical, and moderate-intensity physical activity daily for a period lasting 30 minutes or longer. Periods of physical activity lasting 15 minutes or so during the day can be added together. Doing even more exercise adds more benefit. Therefore, exercising beyond the current recommendations will help individuals with the metabolic syndrome. Sixty minutes or more of continuous or intermittent aerobic activity, preferably daily, will enhance weight loss and weight maintenance. Sedentary leisure activities should be replaced by more active ones, such as brisk walking, jogging, swimming, biking, golfing, and team sports. Preference should be given to 60 minutes of moderate-intensity brisk walking, to be supplemented by other activities, such as multiple short (10 to 15 minutes) bouts of activity (taking walking breaks at work, gardening, or doing household work), using simple exercise equipment (treadmill, cross-trainer) or engaging in resistance training, or engaging in any of the activities listed in the previous sentence.

Exercise has direct metabolic effects with demonstrable benefits to insulin levels, lipoproteins, the fibrinolytic profile, insulin sensitivity, glucose transporters, and lipoprotein lipase upregulation in skeletal muscle as well as fat distribution and blood pressure. Physical training has various effects on the tissues. Skeletal muscle mass increases with changes in the muscle fiber type, increased capillary density, increased glycogen content, redistributed intramyocyte triglycerides, and induction of various enzymes related to oxidative fuel metabolism [33]. Adipose tissue mass also lessens but there is an increased ability to mobilize and utilize lipid fuel (in contrast to carbohydrate fuels).

Effects on Cardiovascular Disease
There is graded relationship of reducing CAD rates with increasing levels of activity. There is substantial evidence of the benefit of exercise on atherosclerotic risk factors, myocardial function, coronary artery size and vasodilatory capacity, vascular tone, and susceptibility to ventricular fibrillation. It is not clear how long the effects of exercise last, but the benefits of college athletic activity are not lifelong unless accompanied by increased physical activity in later years [34].

Physical activity not only prevents but also helps to treat established CVD risk factors, including high blood pressure, insulin resistance, glucose intolerance, elevated triglycerides level, low HDL cholesterol, and obesity, all of which are components of the metabolic syndrome. The beneficial effect of pharmacological therapies is greater than the effects of exercise on CVD risk factors. However, this benefit can be enhanced if exercise is supplemented with appropriate diet and weight loss. In patients with the metabolic syndrome who have elevated level of triglycerides, the effect of exercise on raising the HDL cholesterol level is substantial. Among older people there is no evidence of increased adverse outcome with exercise. Whether exercise training reduces morbidity and mortality in elderly CAD patients is controversial. However, the British Regional Heart Study showed that men with a mean age of 63 years who did light to moderate physical exercise had significantly lower all-cause mortality over 5-year follow-up than did sedentary men [34].

Effects on Components of the Metabolic Syndrome
Physical exercise favorably affects individual components of the metabolic syndrome, although little evidence exists showing that physical activity prevents the metabolic syndrome [35]. However, moderate and vigorous exercise decreases the risk of the metabolic syndrome independently of obesity and other important confounding factors. Men with high cardiorespiratory fitness are nearly two-thirds less likely to develop the metabolic syndrome.

Even low levels of leisure time physical activity (LTPA) tend to decrease the likelihood of developing the metabolic syndrome, and regular and sustained physical activity will improve all the risk factors of the metabolic syndrome.

A meta-analysis found that exercise intervention lowers LDL cholesterol by 5% and triglycerides by 3.7%, and raises HDL cholesterol by 4.6% [36]. Regular exercise such as brisk walking 30 minutes for most days reduces systolic blood pressure by 4 to 9 mm Hg. In a meta-analysis there was an average reduction of 2.6 mm Hg in systolic blood pressure and 1.8 mm Hg in diastolic blood pressure in the normotensive group but a more marked reduction of 7.4 and 5.8 mm Hg, respectively, was found in individuals who had hypertension upon entering into the studies [36]. Regular exercise is associated with a reduction in insulin resistance, glucose intolerance, postprandial hyperglycemia, and hepatic glucose release [37]. In patients with type 2 diabetes, nine trials have found an average reduction of 0.5% to 1% in glycosylated hemoglobin [37]. Physical activity is an important adjunct to diet in weight loss and weight maintenance [34].

Physical activity assists in long-term smoking cessation by increasing the initial quit rate. Cigarette smoking is associated with the metabolic syndrome, the prevalence of which increases with the number of cigarettes smoked. Of the components of the metabolic syndrome, dyslipidemia and abdominal obesity are shown to be the main contributors to this association. The underlying mechanism, however, is not clear.

Obesity and Weight Loss

Q: What are the methods of measuring obesity?
Obesity can be measured by the traditional methods of body mass index (BMI), waist/hip ratio, and waist circumference (WC). These traditional methods of measuring obesity, along with relative weight tables, are important determinants of a variety of CV risk factors, especially hypertension, dyslipidemia, and diabetes. The BMI is measured by weight in kilograms divided by the height in meters squared (kg/m^2). The BMI is now thought to play a secondary role after abdominal obesity in the development of several metabolic processes. To measure WC, locate the top of the right iliac crest. Place a measuring tape in the horizontal plane around the abdomen at the level of the iliac crest. Before reading the tape measure, ensure that the tape is snug but does not compress the skin and is parallel to the floor. Measurement is made at the end of the patient's normal expiration.

Recently, greater WC alone has been found to be related to an increase in CV events, greater fasting insulin, increased insulin resistance in metabolic studies, and increased abdominal fat assessed by current procedures such as computed tomographic scanning.

The BMI and abdominal obesity (WC or waist/hip ratio) are both important determinants of increased CHD and diabetes [38]. Both WC and BMI were independently associated with the presence of CVD in both sexes [39]. The relationship between CVD and WC/BMI occurred worldwide in both lean and obese individuals.

Q: What are the benefits of weight loss?
Weight loss is associated with improvement of several metabolic factors of the metabolic syndrome such as insulin resistance, type 2 diabetes, dyslipidemia, hypertension, hyperuricemia, thrombogenic factors, cytokines, and arterial dysfunction [40]. A 3500-kcal–deficient diet causes >1 lb loss of body weight as a result of oxidation of lean tissue and associated water losses. An energy deficit of 3500 kcal is required to oxidize 1 lb of adipose tissue. Approximately 75% of the weight loss produced by reduced energy intake is composed of adipose tissue and 25% of fat-free mass (FFM) [18]. The majority, if not all, of the loss of fat is caused by a decrease in the size (triglyceride content) of the existing fat cell, not a decrease in the number of fat cells. Also, an energy-deficient diet decreases intramyocellular and intrahepatic lipids. A review of 19 studies found that exercise plus diet caused a 0.1 kg/week greater loss than did diet alone [18]. Weight loss induced by combining physical activity with diet decreases the loss of FFM that occurs when weight loss is caused by diet alone [18]. Intentional weight loss prevents obesity-related risk factors for CHD, such as insulin resistance, type 2 diabetes, dyslipidemia, hypertension, and inflammation. Interestingly, these benefits are observed even with modest weight loss (5% of initial weight), and continue to improve in a monotonic fashion with increasing weight loss [18].

Insulin Resistance and Type 2 Diabetes
Insulin sensitivity improves rapidly after eating an energy-deficit diet, even before significant weight loss is observed, and this benefit continues with weight loss. A weight loss of 5% toward the end of the first year leads to some measurable benefit such as reduced fasting glucose, insulin level, HbA_{1c} level, and dose of oral antidiabetic drugs. Weight loss prevents the onset of type 2 diabetes in high-risk obese individuals.

Dyslipidemia

Weight loss has beneficial effects on the lipid profile such as reduction of LDL cholesterol and triglyceride levels (and increased HDL cholesterol level where weight loss is sustained). The most beneficial effect on lipids is seen during the first 2 months of weight loss, and the effect is related to the percentage of weight loss. To maintain this beneficial effect on triglycerides, sustained weight loss of ≥ 5% is needed, while for LDL cholesterol, ≥ 10% energy-deficit–induced weight loss needs to be sustained [18].

Inflammatory Markers

The decrease in CRP is seen after 3 months to 2 years of weight loss and is directly related to the amount of weight loss, fat mass, and alteration in WC. A decrease in plasma, IL-6, IL-18, P-selectin, and TNF-α has also been observed after weight loss in obese individuals.

Autonomic Nervous System

A 10% increase in body weight is associated with a decline in parasympathetic tone and an increase in heart rate that is associated with increased CV events and mortality. Energy-deficit–induced sustained weight loss is associated with an increase in parasympathetic activity.

Cardiovascular System

Weight loss reduces both systolic and diastolic blood pressure, and the effect is dose-dependent. Energy-deficit-diet–induced weight loss prevents the development of hypertension in obese individuals. It is not well established that weight loss decreases CVD events or CVD mortality in obese individuals, but obesity is associated with increased CVD mortality and is directly related to BMI in both men and women. Also, being overweight in adolescence is associated with a 130% increased risk of CHD mortality in adulthood [18]. Weight variability is also associated with an increased rate of CVD mortality [18]. Obesity, particularly severe obesity, is associated with abnormalities of cardiac structure and function, and these are dependent on the duration of obesity. These abnormalities improve, however, after weight loss in severely obese individuals.

Q: What components of food are important in the treatment of obesity?

Obesity should be managed by weight reduction, by implementing behavioral changes to reduce calorie intake, and by increased physical activity. Diet, physical activity, and behavioral therapy should be initiated when a patient has a BMI ≥ 25.0. The behavioral modifications include an emphasis on improvement of eating habits (e.g., setting goals, planning meals, eating regular meals, reading and interpreting food labels, reducing portion sizes, avoiding binge eating, and self-monitoring). Other important measures include the benefit of social support, stress management, and enforcement of regular exercise program. Professional support from a nutritionist and counselor should be sought. The most common approach for obese/overweight individuals with the metabolic syndrome is a balanced-calorie diet. When the total calorie intake is advised, the patient's current calorie intake should be calculated, taking into account various factors that affect this need, such as an individual's occupation and physical activity level. The daily calorie intake can be calculated by various methods, such as the Harris-Benedict equation, which is a formula that uses the basal metabolic rate (BMR) (which is 1745) and then applies an activity factor to determine the daily energy expenditure. The activity factors are as follows: for a sedentary individual, 1.2; for a lightly active individual, 1.375; for a moderately active individual, 1.55; for a very active individual, 1.725; and for an extra-active individual, 1.9. From this figure should be deducted the number of calories that need to be reduced (or added if the weight is to be gained). This method, however, does not take into account the lean fat; as a result, it underestimates for leaner individuals and overestimates for very fat individuals. An average man requires 2500 kcal/d, while a woman needs 2100 kcal/d.

Energy-Deficit Diet
A low-calorie diet (LCD) provides 800 to 1500 kcal/d, which produces an 8% loss of body weight at 6 months. A very-low-calorie diet (VLCD) provides <800 kcal/d, which produces a 15% to 20% weight loss within 4 months. With VLCDs, the maintenance of weight loss is difficult; therefore, the net outcome at the end of 1 year is similar to that of LCDs. There are also medical problems associated with VLCDs such as diet-induced hypokalemia, dehydration, and gallstones. The first aim of weight loss is to achieve a reduction of approximately 7% to 10% from the baseline total weight during the 6 to 12 months duration of the diet. The Expert Panel on the Identification, Evaluation, and Treatment of Overweight and Obesity in Adults recommend a 500- to 1000-kcal-deficit diet for obese individuals, which will initially produce a loss of 1 to 2 lb (0.45 to 0.9 kg) per week [18]. Therefore, calorie-intake guidelines depend on the initial weight of the individual. The suggested energy and macronutrient composition of the initial reduced calorie diet

should be as follows: body weight 150 to 199 lb, 1000 kcal: body weight 200 to 249 lb, 1200 kcal; 250 to 299 lb, 1500 kcal; 300 to 349 lb, 1800 kcal, and ≥ 350 lb, 2000 kcal. [20]. A balanced-deficit diet provides ≤ 1500 kcal/d.

A more intensive approach should be enforced in the very obese, and these targets are often achieved by weight loss clinics. An alternative approach is to prescribe a very-low-calorie liquid diet, and this treatment requires intensive outpatient medical supervision and the monitoring of electrolytes and liver function. Long-term weight loss has been problematic, as the weight is often regained. Maintenance of a lower weight is just as important as initial weight loss, and that is achieved by proper follow-up and monitoring of patients.

Macronutrient Composition
A low-fat diet is the standard recommendation because even in the presence of sufficient carbohydrate and protein content, a low-fat diet it is known to provide reduced total energy and thus subsequent weight reduction. A low-fat diet may be preferable in some patients but in general is not more effective than an LCD. It has been a subject of interest to find if alterations in the macronutrient content of the diet could enhance weight reduction. With that view in the past, a low-fat diet was advised because the high calorie density of fat could aggravate obesity. But lately, it has been suggested that a high-protein, low-carbohydrate diet can promote weight loss because of the satiety associated with the fat and protein content of food, which is lacking with carbohydrates. This concept is disputed. Also, the data do not support the idea that a high-fat/high-protein/low-calorie intake (Atkins) for long-term maintenance of lower body weight is suitable. There is evidence that after 1 year of consumption of a low-carbohydrate diet, obese individuals show no more weight reduction as compared to those eating a conventional weight-loss diet [11]. Also, high-fat diets are higher in saturated fat and often deficient in other essential dietary components (e.g., fruits, vegetables, and whole grains).

Recently, low-carbohydrate diets have become very popular. As compared to low-fat diets, low-carbohydrates diets produce twice the weight loss, but the overall result at 1 year is almost similar. However, low-carbohydrate diets are more beneficial for serum triglycerides and HDL cholesterol levels as compared to low-fat diets, but low-fat diets are more beneficial for the LDL cholesterol level. Despite these benefits it is not known if these favorable alterations in lipids are associated with an improved CHD outcome.

The type of carbohydrate consumed is also important. Most refined grain products and potatoes have a high GI, while most fruits, legumes, and nonstarchy vegetables have a low GI. No randomized trial has compared the efficacy of a low-fat diet with that of a low-GI diet in weight reduction, but a small study in obese adolescents found that at 1 year the low-GI diet produced a greater decrease in body weight and BMI than did the low-fat diet [4]. The intake of low-energy-density foods may be another approach in weight management. A randomized controlled trial (RCT) found that ad libitum low-fat and low-energy-density food caused modest (1% to 2%) weight loss at 6 months [18]. Portion control has an important place in achieving a calorie-deficit diet. Studies show that using prepackaged prepared meals, either as frozen entrees of mixed foods or liquid-formula meal replacements, improves portion control and can increase weight loss. It is important to draw attention to food labels, recipe modification, healthy cooking and energy intake during meals and snacks.

Pharmacotherapy

Q: What are the roles of pharmacotherapy and surgical intervention?
Drug therapy is indicated for obese individuals with a BMI ≥ 30, and BMI ≥ 27 for patients with obesity-related illnesses and risk factors, and product labels of prescription antiobesity drugs recommend these criteria. Previously, drug therapy was recommended for short-term use only, but now pharmacotherapy may need to be long-term (if not lifelong) due to the risk of weight regain associated with the cessation of drug therapy. All other standard approaches of weight management, such as behavior modification, diet education, and activity counseling, also need to be adhered to. Pharmacotherapy produces weight loss, predominantly by inhibiting appetite, but it may also have a thermogenic effect mediated by stimulation of the sympathetic nervous system. Drugs approved by the FDA for treating obesity are orlistat, sibutramine HCl, phentermine, diethylpropion HCl, benzphetamine HCl, phendimetrazine tartrate, and rimonabant. Only sibutramine and orlistat are approved in the U.S. for long-term use. In the U.K., only orlistat, sibutramine, and rimonabant are approved for the treatment of obesity. Currently, the available pharmaceutical agents have limited utility in the management of obesity. However, they may be successful in some selected patients. Two main groups of antiobesity agents are appetite suppressants and inhibitors of absorption. The appetite suppressant group includes phentermine derivatives (nonadrenergic) and sibutramine. A meta-analysis

found that the average weight loss with pharmaceutical agents for obesity was approximately 4 kg more than with placebo, and no drug or class of drug was clearly superior [42].

Sibutramine
Sibutramine is a β-phenethylamine derivative that inhibits the reuptake of noradrenaline (norepinephrine) and serotonin from nerve terminals. It is classified as a Schedule IV drug in the U.S. It is used as an adjunct in obesity. Sibutramine is taken once a day in the morning, and it reduces appetite in the late evening. Sibutramine reduces food intake by producing early satiety during feeding and by delaying initiation of the next meal. A recent meta-analysis estimated that 1-year treatment with sibutramine produces an average placebo–subtracted weight loss of 4.5 kg [43]. There is also some evidence that sibutramine helps in maintaining the weight loss as well. Sibutramine is more effective when co-prescribed with behavior therapy or dietary advice. An RCT found that weight loss with sibutramine at 1 year was 5 kg, but weight loss doubled when sibutramine was used with behavior therapy, and trebled when sibutramine was used with behavior therapy and dietary therapy in the form of a structured meal plan [44]. Sibutramine causes an improvement in serum triglyceride, total cholesterol, LDL cholesterol, and HDL cholesterol that is in direct proportion to the degree of weight loss. However, the weight loss-induced benefits on blood pressure are either decreased or eliminated. The dose initially is 10 mg daily in the morning, increased to 15 mg if weight loss is less than 2 kg after 4 weeks, but discontinued if weight loss is less than 2 kg after 4 weeks therapy at higher doses.

Side effects and precautions: Constipation, dry mouth, and insomnia are the most common side effects, but sibutramine may also cause hypertension, urinary retention, flushing, blurred vision, and hypersensitivity reactions. Sibutramine causes a dose-related rise in systolic and diastolic blood pressure of 2 to 4 mg Hg and an increase in heart rate of 4 to 6 bpm, usually in the first few weeks. If blood pressure exceeds 145/90 mm Hg, or if systolic or diastolic blood pressure rises more than 10 mm Hg, or if the pulse rate increases by 10 bpm at consecutive visits, the drug should be discontinued. Sibutramine is contraindicated in the patient with uncontrolled hypertension or a history of CAD, congestive heart failure, cardiac arrhythmias, or stroke, and in the patient treated with a monoamine oxidase inhibitor or a selective serotonin reuptake inhibitor. Sibutramine should be discontinued if (1) weight loss after 3 months less than 5% of initial body weight, (2) weight loss stabilizes at less than 5% of initial body weight, (3) or the patient regains 3 kg or more after previous weight loss. In the U.K. sibutramine is not licensed for use for longer than 1 year.

Orlistat

Orlistat, an inhibitor of the gastrointestinal lipase inhibitor, reduces the absorption of dietary fat and is the only agent available in the nutrient inhibitor class. It is used in conjunction with a mildly hypocalorie diet. Maximum malabsorption of fat occurs with 120 mg taken at mealtime, which produces malabsorption of 30% fat consumed in a meal that contains 30% of energy from fat. A recent meta-analysis estimated that orlistat leads to an average placebo-subtracted weight loss of 2.7 kg at 1 year [45]. Overall, the extent of weight loss produced with orlistat seems to be less than that with sibutramine after 1 or 2 years. Weight loss is often reversed after stopping the drug. Orlistat helped in maintaining weight loss produced by dietary means. When dietary therapy is supplemented with orlistat in a patient with obesity and type 2 diabetes treated with sulfonylureas, metformin, or insulin, it produced a ≥ 5% or ≥10% reduction in body weight, two to three times more as compared to that on dietary therapy alone [20]. In the Xanical in the Prevention of Diabetes in Obese Subjects (XENDOS) study, orlistat produced an 11% weight loss as compared to 6% with placebo in the first year and 6.9% vs. 4.1% at the end of 4 years, and also reduced the cumulative 4-year incidence of type 2 diabetes by 37% [46]. Orlistat is associated with improvement in all major CV risk factors, such as blood pressure and insulin sensitivity. It lowers LDL cholesterol, without any substantial effect on triglycerides. The dose is 120 mg taken immediately before, during, or up to 1 hour after each main meal (max. 360 mg daily).

Side effects: Approximately 15% to 30% of patients suffer troublesome oily leakage from the rectum, flatulence, focal urgency, or liquid or oily stools, and 7% complain of fecal incontinence, particularly on initiation of therapy. Other side effects are menstrual irregularities, infections (respiratory, gingivitis, urinary tract), and hypoglycemia. Rarely, rectal bleeding occurs; very rarely diverticulitis, hepatitis, cholelithiasis, or bullous eruptions occur. Malabsorption may cause lowering of blood levels of fat-soluble vitamins, particularly vitamins A, D, and E, but the level remains within the reference range in most patients. For this reason it is advisable that all patients taking orlistat should take one multivitamin supplement at a different time than orlistat. However, orlistat does not affect the absorption of some selected drugs that have narrow therapeutic index, such as warfarin, digoxin, and phenytoin.

Likewise, the absorption of glyburide, the oral contraception pill, furosemide, nifedipine, captopril, and atenolol is not affected. The NICE study has recommended that treatment with orlistat should be continued beyond 6 months only if there is at least a 10% weight loss since the start of treatment.

Rimonabant

Rimonabant was approved by the FDA in April 2006 for weight management. It has recently been approved in some European countries. It is a selective cannabinoid CB_1 receptor antagonist that has been tested in the management of obesity, as well as for treating nicotine dependence. It provides a novel mechanism of action and may be suitable for some patients who do not respond well to other agents and also for co-therapy with other antiobesity agents. Its pharmacokinetic profile seems to be favorable in general. Rimonabant is prescribed in a dose of 20 mg, and with dieting is associated with a 3.9- to 5.4-kg (8.6- to 11.9-lb) greater weight loss as compared with placebo and dieting after 1 year; this is similar to sibutramine in 1 year. However, a 7.4-kg (16.3-lb) weight loss was observed with continuous 2-year treatment in the Rimonabant In Obesity (RIO) RIO–North American Study [47], but this drug was withdrawn from this study due to the frequency of psychiatric symptoms. There is a negligible reduction in systolic blood pressure that ranges from 0.2 to 2.3 mm Hg relative to placebo, but no reduction of diastolic blood pressure was observed. There is a consistent reduction of triglyceride level, ranging from 12% to 16%, and HDL cholesterol improved by 7% to 9%, but no reduction in total cholesterol or LDL cholesterol occurs. In contrast, orlistat is often associated with greater improvement in total cholesterol and LDL cholesterol relative to placebo and less so with improvements in triglycerides and HDL cholesterol [48].

Rimonabant has demonstrated consistent efficacy in weight reduction (and reduction of WC), and the weight loss seems to improve some features of the metabolic syndrome. It decreases the plasma glucose level among individuals with type 2 diabetes. There is no evidence of any significant CV adverse side effects. In fact, most side effects appear to be mild and transient. Rimonabant should not be prescribed for patients with serious psychiatric illness (e.g., severe depression) until the psychiatric condition is well controlled. It is also not recommended for patients on antidepressants. The limitations of rimonabant are as follows [48]: (1) Weight reduction efficacy with rimonabant is not better than with currently available antiobesity drugs. (2) Although it has better smoking quitting rates, the results are not that impressive, and therefore rimonabant is not presently indicated for this purpose. (3) Although features of the metabolic syndrome improve modestly, no reduction in LDL cholesterol occurs. Rimonabant might have systemic action that independently reduces risk factors for the metabolic syndrome.

Surgery

Patients whose BMI is > 40, or between 35 and 40 with one or more comorbid conditions that are components of metabolic syndrome, and who do not respond to dietary modifications or pharmaceutical agents, may be candidates for surgical intervention, such as bariatric surgery. Presently the surgical procedures that are in use are gastric bypass, Roux-en-Y anastomosis, gastroplasty, gastric banding, biliopancreatic diversion, and biliopancreatic diversion with duodenal switch. Of these, gastric bypass accounts for 70% of bariatric operations, and it produces greater weight loss than does the vertical banded gastroplasty. Some components of the metabolic syndrome (e.g., lipid, glucose concentration) improve with weight loss after surgery. The most effective surgical procedure is a vertical banded gastric bypass surgery where weight typically reduces 40% at 1 year and 62% at 5 years [38]. Postoperatively, careful monitoring is required, including monitoring of vitamin and hematological status, strict compliance with specific postoperative dietary instructions, and psychological support. In the U.S., bariatric surgery is increasingly used to treat individuals with morbid obesity. The effectiveness and safety of bariatric surgery in patients with the metabolic syndrome is quite encouraging, with 95% of patients free of the syndrome 1 year after the surgery [3]. There is marked improvement in insulin sensitivity, endothelial function, and low-grade inflammation in weight-losing, morbidly obese patients after bariatric surgery. For further information, go to www.NHLBI.NIH.gov/ and http://www.american heart.org/.

MANAGEMENT OF METABOLIC RISK FACTORS

Dyslipidemia

Q: What are the guidelines for the management of dyslipidemia in the metabolic syndrome?
In the management of dyslipidemia in the metabolic syndrome, weight loss, increased physical activity, and moderate alcohol intake are the first-line interventions. Weight loss in individuals with visceral obesity reduces VLDL-ApoB secretion and

reciprocally upregulates LDL-ApoB catabolism, most likely due to reduced visceral adiposity, increased insulin sensitivity, and decreased hepatic lipogenesis [49]. Weight loss should reduce the BMI to 25, although even a 10% reduction of weight can improve insulin sensitivity. Moderate-intensity physical activity improves insulin sensitivity. Dietary saturated fatty acids should be reduced. There is a decrease in LDL cholesterol on a low-fat diet in individuals with marked insulin resistance [50]. During weight reduction, cholesterol absorption increases in parallel with improvements in glucose metabolism parameters, suggesting that low cholesterol absorption could be an additional feature of the metabolic syndrome [49]. Moreover, subjects with the metabolic syndrome have a low campesterol/cholesterol ratio, indicative of reduced cholesterol absorption. This ratio was inversely correlated with plasma triglyceride, remnant cholesterol, and ApoB48. Increased intake of n-3 fatty acid (6 to 12 g/d) provides a 40% to 80% reduction in serum triglycerides, by an unknown mechanism [49]. Dietary intake of 9 to 12 oz/d of salmon or concentrated fish oil supplements can provide similar benefit [49]. Hyperlipidemia should be treated according to the NCEP ATP-III guidelines [51] (Table 6.1).

Nicotinic Acid (Niacin)

Q: What is the role of nicotinic acid in the treatment of the metabolic syndrome?

Nicotinic acid (niacin) effectively treats all the common lipid derangements; for example, it lowers plasma cholesterol, triglycerides, VLDL, and LDL cholesterol levels, and raises the HDL cholesterol level. Niacin inhibits hormone-sensitive lipase in adipose tissue. It acts by reducing the production of FFAs by inhibition of lipolysis in adipose tissue. It reduces FFA influx in the liver, which reduces the availability of substrate for VLDL synthesis [49]. This mechanism of action was supported by the identification of a G-protein–coupled receptor that is highly expressed in adipose tissue and to which niacin is a high-affinity ligand. The binding of nicotinic acid to its receptor activates a G-protein signal, which reduces the cyclic adenosine monophosphate (cAMP) levels and thus inhibits lipolysis. Thus, the main effect of niacin is to reduce the hepatic output of VLDL, with consequent reductions in intermediate-density lipoprotein (IDL) and LDL. Reduction of VLDL is also associated with reduction of its protein components: apoproteins B, C, and E.

Nicotinic acid is particularly effective in raising HDL by reducing hypertriglyceridemia. It raises HDL cholesterol through the stimulation of the adenosine triphosphate binding cassette A1 (ABCAI)-mediated transfer of cholesterol [49]. It is highly effective in dysbetalipoproteinemia, and reduction in remnant particles of 50% to 60% can occur. Nicotinic acid also reduces lipoprotein (a). Furthermore, it has a weak effect on hepatic cholesterol synthesis. The beneficial pleiotropic effects on parameters of low-grade inflammation and coagulation have been observed with decrease in hsCRP, fibrinogen, and PAI-1. Improvement in the lipid profile in the metabolic syndrome can be achieved by several mechanisms such as decreased secretion and increased catabolism of ApoB, as well as increased secretion and decreased catabolism of ApoA-I. It is also suggested that nicotinic acid directly inhibits the synthesis of ApoB-containing lipoprotein in the liver [49].

Nicotinic acid in the new extended-release (ER) form is a powerful drug for dyslipidemia in the metabolic syndrome. It is associated with few side effects, smoother delivery, and less hyperglycemic effects than the shorter-acting (crystalline) preparation or the sustained-release preparation. It has additional pleiotropic effects on low-grade inflammation. It increases HDL cholesterol by about 10% to 30%, and decreases triglyceride by 20% to 25%, LDL cholesterol by 10% to 25%, FFA by about 20%, and lipoprotein (a) by 10% to 30% [52].

The HDL cholesterol Atherosclerosis Treatment Study (HATS) reported that in patients with CHD who had normal levels of LDL cholesterol, treatment with simvastatin and nicotinic acid resulted in significant modification of LDL cholesterol ($\downarrow$42%) and HDL cholesterol ($\uparrow$26%) [53]. Consequently, the risk of a first cardiovascular event was reduced by >90%. This was comparable with the risk reductions reported by the key statin trials and firmly established HDL cholesterol as a major independent risk factor for CVD. In combination with a statin, nicotinic acid is a valuable therapy that is effective in raising HDL cholesterol and reducing the risk of CHD. Increases in HDL cholesterol may be observed with lower doses (1 g/d). When a switch is made from immediate-release nicotinic acid to extended-release formulations, equivalent doses should not be substituted. Instead, the extended-release regimen should be initiated at a low dose and titrated to the desired effect (Table 6.2).

Side effects: Cutaneous flushing with a prickly feeling is common. Tachyphylaxis to the flushing occurs rapidly, and aspirin is useful in relieving these symptoms. Other skin side effects include pruritus, rash, dry skin, and, rarely, acanthosis nigricans. Gastrointestinal

TABLE 6.2. Dosage of lipid lowering drugs (refer to the prescribing information relevant to your national formulary and guidelines)

Generic name	Daily dose range	Frequency per day
Cholesterol-lowering		
Statins		
Atorvastatin	10–80 mg	1
Fluvastatin	20–40 mg	1
Pravastatin	10–40 mg	1
Simvastatin	10–40 mg	1
Rosuvastatin	5–40 mg	1
Lovastatin	10–80 mg	1
Bile-acid sequestrants		
Cholestyramine	4–16 g	1–4
Colestipol	5–20 g	1–2
Colesevelam	2.6–3.8 g	1–2
Cholesterol absorption inhibitor		
Ezetimibe	10 mg	1
Triglyceride-lowering		
Fibrates		
Gemfibrozil	600 mg	2
Fenofibrate micro	200 mg	1
Benzafibrate	400 mg	3
Ciprofibrate	100 mg	1
Nicotinic acids		
Nicotinic acid (Niacin)	1–2 g	3
Acipimox	600 mg	3
Nicotinic acid crystalline	1.5–3 g	3
Nicotinic acid extended release	1–2 g	1
Nicotinic acid sustained release	1–2 g	1

symptoms are common. More serious but rare side effects include cardiac arrhythmia, and cystic maculopathy leading to vision loss. Rarely, myopathy can occur, with increased creatine phosphate level. Other side effects include elevated uric acid (precipitation of gout), glucose intolerance, and elevated liver enzyme.

Fibrates

Q: What is the role of fibrates in the treatment of the metabolic syndrome and in cardiovascular prevention?
Fibrates are indicated in patients with disorders of triglycerides or HDL. They are suitable for treating hypertriglyceridemia and

mixed hyperlipidemia. They also affect a number of emerging risk factors, including hemostatic and inflammatory markers and indicators of improved vascular wall biology, which may contribute to their CV protective effects. Fibrates reduce hepatic triglyceride synthesis, and peripheral clearance is enhanced. The effect on the liver is believed to be secondary to increased cellular fatty acid catabolism, resulting in inhibition of hepatic VLDL triglyceride synthesis and secretion. The peripheral clearance is enhanced by the increased activity of enzyme lipoprotein lipase through induction of the gene for lipoprotein lipase and repression of the gene for ApoC-III, an important inhibitor of the enzyme. By reducing VLDL triglyceride and subsequently VLDL size, fibrates increase the production of rapidly catabolized LDL. The LDL particles produced from smaller VLDL particles are larger in size and less dense and are better ligands for the LDL receptor. Therefore, fibrate therapy in isolated hypertriglyceridemia may lead to a slight rise of LDL. However, this increase in LDL mass is accompanied by changes in LDL distribution to larger, more buoyant particles that are less atherogenic. Fibrates reduce the level of hsCRP and fibrinogen [54].

Fibrates act on PPARα receptors that are involved in gene expression for ApoC-III and lipoprotein lipase [55]. Through the activation of PPARα, fibrates affect the expression of five key gene-encoding proteins involved in HDL cholesterol metabolism: ApoA-I, ApoA-II, lipoprotein lipase, scavenger receptor-B1 (SR-B1), and ABCA1. Thus, PPARα increases HDL synthesis and affects reverse cholesterol transport by enhancing the efflux of cholesterol from peripheral cells and its uptake by liver. Fibrates have some pleiotropic effects that may add to the complementary benefit to lipid-lowering action in the metabolic syndrome [56]. An increase in the level of HDL cholesterol associated with fibrate therapy is due to enhanced synthetic rates of ApoA-I and ApoA-II, the major protein constituents of HDL cholesterol. Fibrates induce the transcription rates of *A-I* and *A-II* genes through binding of activated PPARα to promoter regions of the gene. High-density lipoprotein cholesterol may also increase secondary to reductions in triglycerides.

Fibrates can be used in combination with anion exchange resins in mixed hyperlipidemia and with nicotinic acid in severe hypertriglyceridemia. In a patient who is at increased risk of CHD, fibrates may be used with statins in mixed hyperlipidemia. It appears that bezafibrate, ciprofibrate, and particularly fenofibrate are most effective in isolated hypercholesterolemia. As for triglyceride-lowering efficacy, there is not much to choose from among different fibrates in mixed lipidemia. In isolated moderate hypertriglyceridemia, ciprofibrate and fenofibrate are quite efficacious, whereas in the type V phenotype, bezafibrate and gemfibrozil are most efficacious. Gemfibrozil is quite effective in type III dyslipidemia. The typical dyslipidemia of type 2 diabetes of low HDL and raised triglycerides would suggest a significant role for fibrates. If a patient has normal total cholesterol with <15% 10-year risk, low HDL, and raised triglycerides, fibrates could be considered as first-line treatment. Fibrates reduce triglycerides by about 30% to 50% and LDL cholesterol by about 10%, and increase HDL cholesterol by 10% to 15%.

Several trials have investigated the potential of fibrates (particularly gemfibrozil) to reduce CV events. The results have varied widely, but are positive with gemfibrozil in the primary prevention Helsinki Heart Study (HHS) [57] and the Veterans Administration HDL Lipoprotein Intervention Trial (VA–HIT) [60]. The VA-HIT was the first study to suggest that raising HDL cholesterol without lowering LDL cholesterol could reduce the cardiovascular risk [58]. The trial compared the fibrate gemfibrozil with placebo in men with dyslipidemia typical of the metabolic syndrome. At 1 year, mean LDL cholesterol remained the same in both groups. However, mean HDL cholesterol levels were 6% higher and mean triglyceride levels were 31% lower in the fibrate group than in the placebo group. These changes in the treatment arm were associated with reductions of 22% and 25% in myocardial infarction and stroke, respectively. This clearly established HDL cholesterol and the interrelated changes in triglycerides as additional major independent cardiovascular risk factors.

The VA-HIT study carried out nuclear magnetic resonance (NMR) spectroscopy to investigate the effects of gemfibrozil on a number of LDL and HDL subclass particles [59]. Despite having no effect on LDL cholesterol, gemfibrozil markedly increased the size of LDL particles and reduced their overall number. The LDL cholesterol levels were unrelated to CHD events, but LDL particle number at baseline and during the trial were strong, independent predictors of a new CHD event. The LDL particle size, in contrast, was not related to CHD events. Total HDL particle numbers of a small HDL particle subclass were increased by gemfibrozil, and on-trial concentrations of both of these HDL particle parameters predicted CHD events. The Diabetes Atherosclerosis Intervention Study (DHIS) found that there was a significant reduction of progression of coronary atherosclerosis in patients prescribed fenofibrate for type 2 diabetes [60].

Side effects: These include gastrointestinal symptoms and skin rash. The most serious side effect is myositis with muscle pain and elevated CPK level. Clofibrate increases the risk of gallstones formation. Fibrates should not be used in renal impairment, as the drug level tends to rise, which increases the propensity to myositis. Similarly, they should be avoided in biliary disease due to an increased risk of gallstones; otherwise the risk is small. They should not be used in hepatic disease. Occasionally, liver enzymes increase. Benzafibrate and fenofibrate increase homocysteine, whereas gemfibrozil does not. Gemfibrozil in combination with statin increases myopathy and rhabdomyosis.

Statins (HMG-CoA Inhibitors)

Q: What is the mode of action of statins?
Statins (3-hydroxyl-3-methylglutaryl coenzyme A [HMG CoA] inhibitors) are specific competitive inhibitors of the enzyme HMG-CoA reductase, the enzyme involved in the rate-limiting step in cholesterol biosynthesis through conversion of HMG-CoA to mevalonate (see Fig. 3.2 in Chapter 3). They act by reducing cholesterol synthesis in the liver (and other cells and increase its catabolism) with upregulation of LDL receptors and a reduction in plasma LDL levels. This pathway is inhibited by approximately 40%. ApoB concentrations tend to be reduced to a similar degree as LDL cholesterol. High-density lipoprotein and ApoA-I enhance the removal and transfer of cholesterol from the arterial wall back to the liver [61]. Statins increase HDL cholesterol and ApoA-I. This increase may be caused by a decrease in the fractional catabolic rate of ApoA-I or increased production of ApoA-I through the action of its promoter, the PPAR receptor [6]. Peroxisome proliferation–activated receptor-γ is expressed at a high level in the adipose tissue and it is activated by dietary fats, eicosanoids, as well as by drugs such as TZDs. Thiazolidinediones reduce serum triglycerides via PPARγ-mediated induction of lipoprotein lipase expression in adipose tissue [61]. Very low density lipoprotein synthesis involves coupling of lipid (triglyceride and cholesterol) to ApoB, helped by microsomal transfer protein. This process may be affected by statins (through inhibition of HMG- CoA reductase), resulting in reduced synthesis of triglycerides.

Pleiotropic Effects
These effects include improvement in endothelial dysfunction, increased nitric oxide bioavailability, an antioxidant effect, antiinflammatory properties, and stabilization of atherosclerotic plaque. These effects may be independent of their lipid-lowering properties. The cardiovascular benefits of statin therapy, which cannot be

explained purely on the basis of reductions of LDL cholesterol levels, and which appear to be unrelated to baseline lipid measurements, are as follows [62]:

- Statins reduce plasma levels of inflammatory markers, independently of their action in lowering lipid levels.
- Statins increase the expression and activity of antiinflammatory mediators and reduce proinflammatory functions in vitro without altering the lipid profile.
- Statins inhibit proatherogenic processes by directly binding to proinflammatory mediators (lymphocytic function associated antigen-1 [LFA-1], T-cell receptors), independent of their action as HMG-CoA reductase.

Hyperlipidemia reduces the bioavailability of nitric oxide (NO). Hence it is imperative that normal NO release be restored, which promotes vasodilation and interferes with various atherogenic pathways, such as platelet adhesion, superoxide formation, expression of adhesion molecules, and smooth muscle cell (SMC) proliferation. Statins increase the expression of endothelial nitric oxide synthase (eNOS), interfering with oxidative stress pathways, and reducing expression of caveolin. Statins enhance NO bioavailability, thus producing favorable effects on endothelial function. This improves vascular function, which interferes with the atherosclerotic pathway, which in turn leads to plaque vulnerability in CAD. Many of the effects of statins beyond lipid metabolism may be related to their distinct lipophilic and physiochemical properties [63]. Statins stimulate production of endothelial NO via an impressive reduction in plasma membrane caveolin levels and by enhancing the agonist-induced association of eNOS and the chaperone heat shock protein Hsp90, resulting in potent eNOS activation. This is indicative of statin's effect on endothelial function by modulating plasma membrane microdomains and caveolin expression.

Statins may also increase the expression of NO by reducing membrane cholesterol levels, and hence by restoring the normal transport of L-arginine [54]. Statins also reduce LDL oxidation, and increase the bioavailability of NO. Certain statins also have an antioxidant effect by direct scavenging of free radical molecules, independently of their effects on lipid metabolism [64]. In the Incremental Decrease in End points through Aggressive Lipid lowering (IDEAL) study, the investigators found that intensive lowering of LDL cholesterol with atorvastatin compared with simvastatin did not result in a significant reduction in the primary outcome of major coronary events [65]. Statins lower LDL cholesterol by 25% to 60%, increase HDL cholesterol by 5% to 10%, and decrease triglycerides by 10% to 30%. Atorvastatin 10 mg reduces LDL cholesterol by 35%, lovastatin 40 mg by 31%, pravastatin 40 mg by 34%, simvastatin 20 to 40 mg by 35% to 45%, and rosuvastatin 5 to 10 mg by 39% to 45%.

Presently there are no studies to substantiate the use of statins in the metabolic syndrome as such. A post hoc analysis of the West Of Scotland Coronary Prevention Study (WOSCOP study), a primary prevention trial in individuals with hypercholesterolemia, considered the incidence of CHD in patients with the metabolic syndrome (according to modified ATP-III criteria). This study found a 30% lower risk for the development of diabetes in the pravastatin group [66]. A 27% reduction of atherosclerotic cardiovascular disease (ASCVD) in the subgroup with the metabolic syndrome was achieved with pravastatin. The Collaborative AtoRvastatin Diabetes Study (CARDS), a multicenter randomized trial, has found that atorvastatin reduced the incidence of myocardial infarction in type 2 diabetes by 37% and stroke by 48% during a 3.9-year follow-up [67]. In the PRavastatin INflammation CRP Evaluation (PRINCE) study pravastatin reduced hsCRP by 17% [68]. Aggressive LDL cholesterol lowering by atorvastatin even decrease hsCRP by 42% vs. 9.6% with placebo [69].

Safety
The side effects of statins are relatively mild and often transient, such as gastrointestinal symptoms, headaches, and rash. The most important side effect is an asymptomatic increase in hepatic transaminase, but myopathy can occur. The incidence of hepatic transaminase rise is up to 1%, which is dose dependent, similar to all statins, and often occurs during the first 3 months of therapy. The reported incidence of myopathy is 0.1% to 0.2% with statins. The side effect of myopathy occurs during the first few weeks to more than 2 years after initiation of therapy, and the clinical presentation of myopathy is broad, varying from muscle ache to severe pain and restriction of mobility and increased creatine kinase (CK) levels in the blood. However, the clinical signs may arise in the absence of a CK increase. Fatal rhabdomyolysis has been reported at the rate of <1 death per 1 million prescriptions for all presently available statins. Statins require extreme precaution and monitoring of CK levels. The factors that increase myopathy include increasing age, female gender, renal or liver disease, diabetes mellitus, hypothyroidism, debilitating status, surgery, trauma, excessive alcohol intake, heavy exercise, uncontrolled dose of niacin or fibrate, and concurrent use of certain drugs such as cyclosporine, protease inhibitors, or drugs metabolized through cytochrome P-450 (CYP). Patients should be advised to watch for early warning symptoms.

Except for pravastatin, all other statins undergo extensive microsomal metabolism by the CYP isoenzyme system. Approximately 50% of all drugs currently available in clinical practice are biotransformed in the liver primarily by the CYP450 3A4, including lovastatin, simvastatin, and atorvastatin, whereas CYP2C9 enzyme is primarily responsible for metabolizing fluvastatin, the CYP34A and CYP2C8 contributing to a lesser extent. However, rosuvastatin is not extensively metabolized but has some interaction with the CYP2C9 enzyme. These differences in the metabolic properties of different statins may account for the variation in their plasma levels and increased drug interactions.

Cholesterol Absorption Inhibitors
Ezetimibe is a cholesterol absorption inhibitor that provides an additional 18% reduction in LDL cholesterol over that seen with statins. Given that when statin doses are doubled, an average 6% further LDL cholesterol reduction is observed, then there is room for a low-dose statin/ezetimibe combination (now available). Ezetimibe is particularly useful in combination (but can be used alone) with statins, where LDL cholesterol is not reduced sufficiently with statins or where statins are not well tolerated or contraindicated. The tolerability and safety profiles are excellent.

Combination Therapy
Combination therapy is indicated when monotherapy has failed. The combinations in the metabolic syndrome may involve statin/fibrate, statin/nicotinic acid, and statin/fish oil. The former two have been reported to increase the risk of drug-induced myopathy and rhabdomyosis, and such combinations are safe. Low or moderate doses of statin (10 to 40 mg/d) with fenofibrate (200 mg/d) or bezafibrate (400 mg/d) are thought to be effective and safe for the treatment of atherogenic dyslipidemia. The safety of the combination may depend on their use in low or intermediate doses. The ezetimibe and simvastatin combination is now available.

Diabetes

Insulin Sensitizers

Metformin

Q: What are the therapeutic benefits of metformin in the metabolic syndrome and cardiovascular disease?
The reduction of insulin resistance at every stage of evolution of type 2 diabetes from compensatory hyperinsulinism to overt type

2 diabetes improves glucose metabolism. Additionally, by reducing insulin resistance, the severity and number of components of the metabolic syndrome are reduced. Metformin increases insulin-mediated glucose disposal in skeletal muscle, and decreases elevated hepatic glucose production that is associated with fasting hyperglycemia. This effect is due primarily to a decrease in gluconeogenesis, but glycogenolysis may also contribute to some extent. It does not have any direct effect on β cells of the pancreas and does not affect insulin secretion directly, but may do so through its role in altering plasma glucose levels. Metformin has not been shown to increase adiponectin (unlike TZDs), but it reduces FFA secretion, decreases intestinal absorption of glucose, enhances peripheral glucose uptake, and increases lipid oxidation in some.

Peak plasma concentration reaches 1 to 2 µg/mL at 1 to 2 hours after an oral dose of 500 to 1000 mg. It has a plasma half-life of 1.5 to 4.9 hours. The peak plasma levels obtained with a 1000- and 2000-mg dose of the extended-release form (now available) were 1.1 and 1.8 µg/mL, respectively. Metformin does not undergo hepatic metabolism or biliary excretion, but is rapidly cleared by the kidneys (90% in 1 hour); therefore, the accumulation of drug in the body does not occur in the presence of normal renal function.

The United Kingdom Prospective Diabetes Study (UKPDS) [70] and the registration studies in the U.S. provide good evidence of the efficacy of metformin. In the registration studies, metformin, when used in obese, type 2 diabetic patients as monotherapy, with a baseline HbA_{1c} of 8.3% and fasting plasma glucose (FPG) of 240 mg/dL (13.32 mmol/d) for 29 weeks, lowered the HbA_{1c} to 1.8% and the mean FPG to 58 mg/dL (3.32 mmol/d). The glucose-lowering effect was greatest with the highest HbA_{1c} and FPG levels [71]. The efficacy of metformin and sulfonylureas appear to be the same, though they act through different mechanisms. Glycemic control, therefore, does not improve if the sulfonylurea is replaced by metformin or vice versa. Combining the two, however, is addictive.

Metformin has many favorable effects on the patient with the metabolic syndrome. A patient taking metformin has some degree of anorexia, and a mean loss of weight of 2 to 3 kg caused primarily by decreased adipose tissue, particularly visceral adiposity. Metformin reduces obesity, particularly central obesity; improves fibrinolysis by decreasing PAI-1; and likely improves the insulin level. Metformin can lower the total cholesterol by up to 5%, triglycerides by 16%, and LDL cholesterol by 8%, with modest increases in HDL cholesterol of 2% to 5%, according to the UKPDS [70]. The beneficial effects of metformin on various derangements were confirmed by the UKPDS in 1998 [72]. Metformin was the only drug in this mega-trial that significantly reduced CV events

[70]. Glibenclamide and insulin also had comparable effects on HbA$_{1c}$ but lacked this CV protection. The reason for this may have been its favorable effect on overweight patients. Metformin also has a favorable effect on most, if not all, components of the metabolic syndrome, in which it is likely to reduce macrovascular complications associated with this syndrome. In the UKPDS, metformin reduced the risk of myocardial infarction and diabetes-related deaths when used in obese type 2 diabetic patients.

Metformin is the drug of choice for overweight and obese type 2 diabetics. However, metformin is equally effective in normal-weight individuals and is now used extensively as a first-line monotherapy for type 2 diabetes, inadequately controlled by diet, exercise, or lifestyle management. It can be used in the elderly provided that renal function is normal. Metformin can be used in combination with any other class of oral antidiabetic drugs and with insulin. Extended-release metformin is safe and efficacious as an immediate-release formulation (Table 6.3).

Side effects: The most troublesome side effects are dose-related gastrointestinal symptoms in 5% to 20% patients, such as metallic taste, anorexia, nausea, abdominal pain, and diarrhea. Lactic acidosis is very rare (3 per 100,000 patient-years), and almost always occurs in cases in which metformin is contraindicated (e.g., impaired renal failure and illnesses that predispose to impaired renal function). Cimetidine can increase the plasma metformin concentration. Metformin should be temporarily discontinued when the patient is undergoing a radiological procedure involving administration of iodinated contrast material as it can interfere with renal function.

Contraindications: These include (1) impaired renal function: plasma creatinine ≥ 1.5 mg/dL for men and ≥ 1.4 mg/dL for women or a creatinine clearance < 60 mL/min; (2) patients with congestive heart failure (CHF) on drug management; (3) age ≥ 80 years, unless creatinine clearance indicates normal renal function; and (4) liver disease, sepsis, or other acute illness.

An extended release formulation is approved for patients who are 17 years old or older. Metformin is also available as a combination product with glipizide, glyburide, or rosiglitazone. A fixed-dose combination of rosiglitazone plus metformin is available in the U.S. and Europe

Thiazolidinediones (TZDs)

Q: What is the role of TZDs in the treatment of insulin resistance and diabetes?

Thiazolidinediones (TZDs) were discovered in 1970s. They delay or prevent the development of type 2 diabetes in an insulin-resistant

TABLE 6.3. Oral antidiabetic agents (refer to the prescribing information relevant to your national formulary and guidelines)

Oral drugs	Dose range mg/d (max. single dose)	Usual maintenance (mg)
Insulin Secretogogues		
Sulfonylureas		
Chlorpropamide	100–500 (750)	250–750 od[b]
Tolbutamide	500–3000	divided
Glibenclamide	2.5–15 (15)	1.25–15 od[b]
Glyburide[a]	1.5–12	0.75–12 od or[b]
Glipizide	2.5–25 (15)#	5–15 od
Glipizide-GIT	5–20	od/bid
Glimepiride	1–8 (6)	1–4 od
Gliclazide	40–320 (160)	Single or divided
Gliclazide MR	30–120	od
Gliquidone	45–180 (60)	Single or divided
Meglitinide		
Repaglinide	1.5–12 (4)	0.5–4, 30 min before meals tid
Nateglinide	180–360 (180)	120, 15–30 min before meals tid
Dipeptidyl Peptidase-4 Inhibitor		
Sitagliptin	100 mg	100 mg
Insulin sensitizers		
Metformin	500–3000**	500–3000 od
Metformin ER	1000–2000	1000–2000 od
Thiazolidinedione		
Rosiglitazone	2–8 (8)	4–8 od
Pioglitazone	15–45 (45)	15–30 od
α-Glucosidase inhibitors		
Acarbose*	150–300 (100)	50–100 tid
Miglitol*	150–300 (100)	50 tid
Voglibose	0.1–0.2	0.1 tid

*Initial dose 25 mg, after 2 weeks, start off with breakfast, after a few weeks 25 mg with midday meal.
**Maximum effect with 1750–2000 mg/d.
#Usual maximum dose in U.S. is 40 mg/d, but little benefit with more than 15 to 20 mg/d.
[a]Micronized formulation of glibendamide.
[b]Divided doses: od, once a day; bid, twice a day; tid, three times a day.

individual. Presently, TZDs are used to treat both insulin resistance and type 2 diabetes. Thiazolidinediones, like metformin and acarbose, are antihyperglycemic rather than hypoglycemic, and require the presence of adequate quantities of insulin to generate an appropriate glucose-lowering effect. They are not a substitute for the absence of insulin. Peroxisome proliferation–activated receptor-γ is the receptor to which TZDs bind and they improve insulin sensitivity by stimulating PPARγ. As discussed earlier, PPARs are of three subtypes—PPARα, PPARγ, and PPARβ/δ—which have distinct actions. All three bind to specific response elements of genes that have a central role in the storage and catabolism of fatty acids. Peroxisome proliferation–activated receptor-α is present in high concentrations in the liver and is activated by fibrates, which are pharmacological ligands for the receptor [71]. Peroxisome proliferation–activated receptor-δ/β is ubiquitous, and its activation by specific pharmacological ligands has a strong affect on lipoprotein metabolism. The major pharmacological action of TZDs in vivo are to increase insulin-mediated glucose uptake (thereby decrease insulin resistance) in muscle and to increase adipogenesis. Peroxisome proliferation–activated receptor-γ receptor is primarily expressed in adipose tissue, being >10-fold higher than in muscle. Despite this, the major insulin sensitizing activity occurs in muscles. Thiazolidinediones operate in association with the retinoid receptor to increase transcription of certain insulin-sensitive genes, which include lipoprotein lipase (LPL), fatty acyl- CoA synthase, and the insulin-sensitive glucose transporter, GLUT-4. Stimulation of PPARγ by TZDs enhances adipose differentiation and lipogenesis, and increases the local effects of insulin.

Thiazolidinediones increase body fat with redistribution of regional obesity; reduction of intraabdominal fat depots and an increase in subcutaneous fat improve insulin sensitivity despite facilitating adipogenesis (lipogenesis). They are insulin sensitizers that have additional benefits on dyslipidemia and hyperglycemia.

Stimulation of lipogenesis via PPARγ reduces not only circulating FFAs (by 20% to 25%) but also TNF-α, resistin, and leptin, released from adipose tissue. Reduction of FFA facilitates glucose uptake by muscle and insulin sensitive adipocytes, and reduces gluconeogenesis in the liver by correcting the glucose–fatty acid cycle. These drugs also increase the release of adiponectin, which is associated with increased hepatic insulin sensitivity [72]. Both pioglitazone and rosiglitazone reduce hsCRP and other inflammatory markers (e.g., IL-6) and PAI-1. Thiazolidinediones are effective when used as monotherapy but also have a synergistic effect when used in combination with biguanides (metformin), sulfonylureas, glinids, or exogenous insulin.

The PROspective pioglitAzone Clinical Trial In macro Vascular Events (PROACTIVE) trial demonstrated a strong trend toward decreasing CV outcome with pioglitazone [73]. The primary end point of time from randomization to the occurrence of new macrovascular events or death was not statistically significant. However, the small improvement in the secondary end point of all-cause mortality, nonfatal myocardial infarction (MI), or stroke was statistically significant. The interpretation of this finding has been controversial [74]. However, PROACTIVE is the only randomized trial to assess the effects of pioglitazone on CV events.

Rosiglitazone and pioglitazone are rapidly well absorbed when taken orally. Both these drugs are extensively metabolized in the liver by CYP450 isoenzymes (rosiglitazone by CYP2C8 and CYP2C9, and pioglitazone by CYP2C8 and CYP3A4) and some other isoenzymes. The plasma half-life of rosiglitazone is 3 to 4 hours and that of pioglitazone and its active metabolites is 16 to 24 hours. Unlike metformin, both drugs are safe in the patient with impaired renal function.

For patients who are poorly controlled with diet and physical activity, rosiglitazone prescribed at 4 and 8 mg daily decreased HbA_{1c} and FPG by 1.2% and 58 mg/dL and by 1.5% and 76 mg/dL, respectively. Pioglitazone at 15 and 45 mg daily reduced HbA_{1c} and FPG by 1.0% and 39 mg/dL and by 1.6% and 65 mg/dL, respectively [71]. Both these drugs have similar efficacy, improve insulin sensitivity, decrease plasma insulin, and improve dyslipidemia associated with insulin resistance (e.g., raise HDL, reduce triglycerides to some extent). Pioglitazone, in particular, has a beneficial effect on dyslipidemia associated with type 2 diabetes, including increasing HDL cholesterol and lowering triglycerides. Additionally, the assessment of the antiatherogenic effects of pioglitazone has shown that the composition of lipid subfraction also improves with pioglitazone, with reduced levels of atherogenic small, dense LDL particles in type 2 diabetics. Unlike pioglitazone, rosiglitazone produced a small increase in LDL cholesterol level (and reduced triglycerides only if they were raised), probably due to shift in the characteristics of LDL particles from small, dense, very atherogenic particles to large, buoyant, less atherogenic particles and not to a real increase in the number of particles. Pioglitazone, on the other hand, does not raise LDL cholesterol and also reduces triglycerides generally. The glycemic effect is similar. Hence, this group of drugs has many potential cardioprotective effects. A recent trial concluded that pioglitazone has a more favorable effect than rosiglitazone in raising HDL cholesterol and in lowering triglycerides [75].

Compared to placebo, pioglitazone monotherapy significantly decreased fasting serum triglyceride level (-16%, $p = .0178$) and increased HDL cholesterol level (12.6%, $p = .0065$).

Markers of inflammation, coagulation, and thrombosis, blood pressure, and the urinary albumin/creatinine ratio (a measure of microalbuminuria) have all been improved with TZDs. Both rosiglitazone and pioglitazone significantly improve the albumin/creatinine ratio, accompanied by a reduction in blood pressure, in patients with type 2 diabetes compared with comparator oral agents. Thiazolidinediones reduce plasma PAI-1 levels, which reduce the inhibition of fibrinolysis.

Side effects: Side effects include fluid retention, increased plasma volume, reduced hematocrit, reduced hemoglobin (Hb), peripheral edema, congestive heart failure (CHF), and weight gain (similar in magnitude to that from sulfonylurea), typically 1 to 4 kg and stabilizing over 6 to 12 months. The weight gain is due to fluid retention and an increase in adipose tissue. The edema responds unsatisfactorily to loop diuretics and angiotensin-converting enzyme (ACE) inhibitors. Thiazolidinediones are contraindicated in CHF. The Hb should be checked before commencing TZDs, as a reduction of up to 1 g/dL may occur during therapy.

It may take 2 to 3 months for these drugs to show their full effect. They can be used in the elderly. Alanine aminotransferase (ALT) should be tested before commencing the treatment and checked periodically. While switching oral combinations to include TZDs, triple therapy (e.g., metformin, sulfonylureas or meglitinide, and TZD) is often recommended while the dose of TZD is titrated up and one of the other agents titrated down. Rosiglitazone is licensed to be used in triple therapy in Europe.

Q: What is the clinical evidence for the beneficial effects of PPARγ agonist in the prevention of atherosclerosis?
The TZDs are specific, high-affinity agonists of the PPARγ. Peroxisome proliferation–activated receptor-γ is a transcription cofactor that modifies expression of the various genes responsible for the encoding of proteins that are involved in lipid and glucose metabolism in homeostasis. The PPARγ agonists act upon adipocytes to modulate insulin-acting signaling, cytokine production, and FFA metabolism, and thereby increase insulin sensitivity. Since insulin exerts a variety of its effects on vascular homeostasis, resistance to insulin leads to various vascular complications. These complications may develop during the prediabetic state and subsequently on clinical manifestation of type 2 diabetes, and they lead to further enhancement of

atherosclerosis and CHD. Peroxisome proliferation–activated receptor-γ is expressed in endothelial cells, vascular smooth muscle cells, and inflammatory cells, which are incriminated in atherosclerosis (e.g., macrophages and T cells). Therefore, it can be said that the PPARγ receptor controls various cellular activities and thereby has a protective effect on CVD associated with insulin resistance [76].

Endothelial Dysfunction

For descriptive purpose, the various effects of TZDs can be discussed during the various stages of atherosclerotic process. Endothelial cells play a crucial role in the regulation of homeostasis by expressing various vasoactive substances. Endothelial dysfunction (ED) in type 2 diabetes characteristically manifests an imbalance in the opposing actions of vasodilator nitric oxide (NO) and the vasoconstriction peptide endothelin-1 (ET-1). Endothelin-1 acts on two types of receptors: ET_A and ET_B. In vascular smooth muscle cells, activation of both receptors causes vasoconstriction, while in endothelial cells, ET_B receptor causes vasodilation [76]. Infused insulin stimulates both NO and ET-1 activity in the skeletal muscle of healthy individuals. However, in type 2 diabetes there is an increased level of circulatory ET-1 and ET_A-dependent vasoconstrictor activity. Endothelial dysfunction and progressive inflammation have been linked to microalbuminemic renal damage in individuals with diabetes. They also have increased urinary ET-1. This shows that increased activity of ET-1 may play a role in vasoconstriction, which characterizes ED in patients with diabetes.

Endothelial dysfunction occurs during the very early stages of atherosclerosis. The evidence of ED in individuals with type 2 diabetes can be shown by measurement of the levels of adhesion molecules (e.g., vascular cell adhesion molecule-1 [VCAM-1], intercellular adhesion molecule-1 [ICAM-1], and E-selectin). Thiazolidinediones have been shown to inhibit their production by activated endothelial cells, hence reducing monocyte/macrophage recruitment. In a nondiabetic individual with CHD, TZD therapy appreciably reduced E-selectin, von Willebrand factor (vWF), and fibrinogen levels, but there was no alteration in ICAM-1 or VCAM-1 [77]. Thiazolidinediones in type 2 diabetes significantly reduced the plasma CRP level.

It is interesting to evaluate the relationship between insulin resistance and vascular homeostasis at the arterial cellular level.

After binding to its receptor, insulin acts via two independent pathways:

1. The phosphatidylinositol (PI)-3-kinase pathway: This pathway appears to be responsible for most of the metabolic actions of insulin, and by this route insulin induces endothelial NO synthase, and thus stimulates the release of NO [76]. Type 2 diabetics show significant resistance to the activation of this route. Individuals with type 2 diabetes manifest profound resistance to the activation of this pathway.

2. Mitogen-activated protein (MAP) kinase: Activation of MAP kinase mediates insulin's stimulation of cell proliferation, ET-1, PAI-1, and adhesion molecules (e.g., E-selectin, VCAM-1). This route is not suppressed by insulin resistance and type 2 diabetes, and may even be increased in this situation. This apparent "selective insulin resistance" may explain the defective vascular homeostasis associated with atherosclerosis with type 2 diabetes [76]. The above reasoning is suggestive that any drug that reduces ET-1 activity or increases NO activity may alter favorably this imbalance responsible for ED in type 2 diabetes. Thiazolidinediones seem to meet these criteria. They inhibit thrombin- and LDL-induced ET-1 secretion in vitro by interfering with the activator protein–1 signaling pathway [78]. Pioglitazone (unlike glibenclamide and voglibose) reduces urinary levels of ET-1 by more than half and urinary albumin secretion by two thirds [76]. In type 2 diabetes the circulating level of ET-1 and of ET_A-dependent vasoactivator activity is enhanced, which may in turn be responsible for ED and progressive inflammation.

Thiazolidinediones also stimulate NO production in a dose-dependent fashion by inducing the enzyme that catalyzes NO production and cNOS via both PPARγ-dependent and PPARγ-independent pathways [79]. Nitric oxide has various beneficial effects. It acts as a vasodilator, and protects against endothelial dysfunction and atherosclerosis. It also inhibits expression by endothelial cells such as monocyte adhesion molecules and chemokines so that they are not available for recruitment, which is necessary for atherosclerosis.

Leucocyte Chemotaxis and Foam Cell Formation
Peroxisome proliferation–activated receptor-γ seems to modulate the leukocyte and monocyte chemotaxis induced by activated endothelial cells. Thiazolidinediones appear to decrease macrophage/monocyte-recruitment, suppress the release of chemokine (monocyte

chemotactic protein-1 [MCP-1]) and expression of adhesion molecules (VCAM-1 and ICAM), and inhibit activation of lymphocytes [76]. The level of soluble CD40 ligand (sCD40L) is raised in diabetes (both type 1 and type 2), and TZDs reduce the inflammatory effects of sCD40L. CD40 receptor and its proinflammatory cytokine, sCD40L, have important roles in atherosclerosis. This ligand plays an important role in atherosclerosis by its atherogenic effects on endothelial cells, vascular smooth muscle cells, macrophages, and lymphocytes in vitro, including the induction of chemokines, cytokines, matrix-degrading metalloproteinases (MMPs), and growth factors, and expression of adhesion molecules [80]. Further, the hindrance of CD40/sCD40L signaling decreases the composition of atheroma and stabilizes atherosclerotic plaques in mice [80]. These plaques are more likely to be oxidized as opposed to larger, more buoyant particles. They are associated with an increased incidence of myocardial infarction.

Peroxisome proliferation–activated receptor-γ regulates lipid homeostasis by regulating the uptake of glycated LDL and triglyceride-rich proteins by macrophages, and therefore affect the formation of foam cells and fatty streaks [81], an initial process in atherosclerosis. It also enhances the efflux of cholesterol from macrophages. A recent study has found that the uptake of oxidized LDL by vascular macrophages is mediated in vivo by the increased expression of cell surface CD36 protein, which is caused, in turn by insulin resistance in macrophages arising from the depletion of insulin receptors and phosphorylation of IRS-2 [82]. Thiazolidinediones reverse the oxidized LDL by vascular macrophages, CD36 activation, and insulin resistance in this model [82].

As discussed elsewhere, TZDs also have a favorable quantitative effect on LDLs that may inhibit the formation of foam cell. They also reduce LDL oxidation. Thiazolidinediones also appreciably reduce the fraction of small, dense LDLs in obese individuals and nonobese type 2 diabetics with CAD and insulin resistance [76]. As a result, TZDs also decrease lipoprotein lipase activity in macrophages, and the macrophages' ability to take up glycated LDL and triglyceride is reduced. Thiazolidinediones reduce the progression of early atherosclerotic remodeling in type 2 diabetic patients.

Plaque Progression, Stability, and Rupture
In this stage of atherosclerosis, migration and proliferation of vascular smooth muscle cell occurs. Peroxisome proliferation–activated receptor-γ activation inhibits chemoattractant-induced migration of vascular smooth muscle cell [83]. Thiazolidinediones have various

antiinflammatory actions, including inhibition of cytokines produced by monocytes (e.g., IL, TNF) and lymphocytes (e.g., T-helper-1 [Th1] cytokines) [8]. Thiazolidinediones may stabilize plaques by inhibiting the production of MMP-9 by macrophages and monocytes and by reducing platelet aggregation. Furthermore, administration of TZDs with simvastatin also significantly reduced MMP-2 activity. These findings suggest that TZDs should be used early in the treatment of patient with type 2 diabetes to achieve adequate CV risk management and glycemic control.

Thiazolidinediones reduce the CRP level independent of any effect on the blood sugar level. Pioglitazone improves coagulation and thrombosis parameters in type 2 diabetics independent of glycemic control; and platelets, von Willebrand factor (a marker of endothelial dysfunction), and PAI-1 are reduced, whereas antithrombic-III and fibrinogen are increased [84]. Pioglitazone also reduces the pulse wave velocity (a marker of vascular damage and a predictor of mortality in diabetes). Pioglitazone also reduces carotid intima-media wall thickness (an early sign of atherosclerotic change) in type 2 diabetes.

Q: What is the mode of action of a-glucosidase inhibitors and what are their indications?

α-Glucosidase inhibitors only delay (but do not decrease) postprandial carbohydrate digestion and lower postprandial plasma glucose excursions by delaying the absorption of polysaccharides and disaccharides in the intestinal border. This gives the β cells more time to match the insulin response to subsequent glucose demands. α-Glucosidase inhibitors slow the process of carbohydrate digestion by competitively inhibiting the activity of α-glucosidase enzyme located in the brush border of the enterocytes lining the intestinal villi. Complex carbohydrates are broken down by amylases in the small intestine into oligosaccharides. Oligosaccharides are poorly absorbed; therefore, they need to be broken down into monosaccharides to facilitate rapid absorption. This breakdown of oligo- into monosaccharide occurs in the brush border of enterocytes by α-enzymes (glucoamylase, sucrose, maltase, dextrinase, and isomaltase). The digestion of complex carbohydrates normally occurs in the distal duodenum and proximal jejunum. The mechanism of action of different α-glucosidase inhibitors is similar but not identical. Acarbose binds to glucoamylase, maltase, sucrose, and dextrinase. Voglibose inhibits most α-glucosidase enzymes but has a weaker effect than acarbose at inhibiting sucrose and has a small effect on pancreatic amylase. Miglitol has greater activity than acarbose on isomaltase. Unlike acarbose, miglitol has no effect on pancreatic amylase. Acarbose and voglibose, unlike miglitol (which has more effect), do not interfere with glucose absorption through the intestinal sodium-dependent glucose transporter. Acarbose also slightly reduces the activity of α–amylase. α-Glucosidase inhibitors are effective only if the diet contains at least 40% to 50% carbohydrates.

Acarbose, when used as monotherapy in a diet-treated type 2 diabetic, produces a mean decrease in the peak postprandial rise in plasma level of 54 mg/dL (3.00 mmol/L) and is associated with a mean decrease in HbA_{1c} of 0.9%. The mean decrease of FPG is approximately 24 mg/dL (1.38 mmol/L). Voglibose is reported to lower the mean HbA_{1c} by between 0.3% and 0.7% [71]. This group of drugs when used with sulfonylurea or insulin may help in glycemic control while reducing the risk of hypoglycemia. α-Glucosidase inhibitors are indicated as adjunctive monotherapy for type 2 diabetes in patients who are inadequately controlled with lifestyle measures. They can also be used with other classes of oral antidiabetic agents or insulin. Miglitol (not available in the U.K.) and acarbose are currently approved for monotherapy (as also initial therapy) and in combination with sulfonylureas, insulin, metformin, and the TZDs. Because these drugs reduce postprandial hyperglycemia, they can be used as first-line monotherapy in patients who have only slightly raised basal glucose concentration or more severe postprandial hyperglycemia. Other beneficial effects include slight weight loss (<1.0 kg), a slight reduction of postprandial triglycerides, and an increase in glucagon-like peptide-1 [85]. In a meta-analysis of studies in type 2 diabetes of at least 1-year duration, acarbose improved several components of metabolic syndrome: overweight, hypertension, and hypertriglyceridemia. There was also a reduction of the incidence of MI by 65% [86]. The Study TO Prevent Non–Insulin-Dependent Diabetes Mellitus (STOP-NIDDM) trial confirms the beneficial the role of both acarbose and metformin in IGT and the metabolic syndrome [87].

Side effects: These include gastrointestinal, abdominal discomfort, flatus, and diarrhea due to excess carbohydrates reaching the colon, where they are fermented. Acarbose and voglibose rarely produce jaundice. They are contraindicated in chronic gastrointestinal disease. Those individuals suffering from gastrointestinal disturbance with metformin are not suitable candidates. Alanine aminotransferase should be checked periodically, and if there is rise, the dose of α-glucosidase inhibitor should be reduced until the ALT is normalized. Since this drug is excreted in urine (unchanged), it is contraindicated in severe renal disease. However, it does not cause weight gain.

Secretogogues

Q: How do new and old secretogogues differ in clinical use?
Sulfonylureas are indicated in patients with hyperglycemia whose blood glucose is not controlled with diet and lifestyle changes. They are not the first choice for treatment, but they may find a place in combination with other drugs when there is difficulty in attaining adequate glycemic control. They stimulate insulin secretion through a direct effect on the pancreatic β cells. These drugs bind to a specific receptor on the β cells of pancreas that increases the effect on glucose lowering resulting from a closure of the adenosine triphosphate (ATP)-dependent potassium channel (K_{ATP}) in the plasma membrane of the β cell. There has been concern about whether sulfonylureas have an adverse effect on cardiovascular system. The concern relates to closure of the potassium channel, because this channel may play a role in cardiac tissue in coronary vasodilation. The closing of the potassium pump increases calcium influx into the myocardial cell, thus promoting coronary artery vasodilation. It has been suggested that this impairment of the potassium pump impairs coronary artery vasodilation during acute ischemic events. The difference in the insulin secretory characteristic depends on this binding to the sulfonylurea receptor (SUR-1) subunit.

Sulfonylureas
All insulin secretogogues including newer nonsulfonylurea repaglinide and nateglinide act by binding to the SUR-1 subunit of the K_{ATP} channels, causing them to close. Sulfonylureas do not correct early insulin deficiency (as seen in type 2 diabetes), but their primary action is to increase the late stage of insulin secretion. This mode of action gives rise to the propensity of late postprandial and fasting hypoglycemia. There is also concern about sulfonylureas' prolonged effect, which may give rise to desensitization, with reduction of their therapeutic effects. The efficacy of sulfonylureas depends on good β-cell function and the absence of antibodies to glutamic acid decarboxylase or islet cells for their efficacy. Their efficacy is almost similar to that of other preparations, although glimepiride may be slightly more effective. On average there is a 1.5% to 2% reduction in HbA_{1c}, with entry (initial HbA_{1c}) greater than 9%. Generally, the reduction is greater when FPG is highest. This class of drugs does no preserve β-cell function.

Sulfonylureas are metabolized in the liver and excreted through the kidneys. Therefore, hypoglycemia is more likely to occur in patients with renal insufficiency except in those taking glipizide, as its hepatic metabolites are not active. Glyburide may cause more hypoglycemia due to its significant suppression of gluconeogenesis and its longer duration of action. Therefore, in patients more likely to suffer hypoglycemia (due to declining renal function, as in the elderly), shorter-acting glipizide is the preferred alternative. Sulfonylureas induce tighter glycemic control and is useful in reducing microvascular complications but not macrovascular complications (e.g., MI) due to potassium channel interference. Chlorpropamide can cause significant hyponatremia and is not presently recommended due to its side effects. As glibenclamide is a long-acting drug, it should be avoided. Sulfonylureas can be used in combination with any different class of oral antidiabetic drugs and have also been used with bedtime insulin, though it is not a normal practice in the U.K.

Glyburide is most effective in controlling hyperglycemia during the first year or two, but their effect gradually declines to almost nil in 4 to 5 years. Glipizide is available in both short-acting and extended-release formulation (glipizide-gastrointestinal/therapeutic system [GIT]). Glimepiride is the newest sulfonylurea and may have an insulin-sparing effect and lower rates of hypoglycemic attacks. Its efficacy is comparable to that of glyburide. Glipizide-GIT has an improved metabolic profile compared to the immediate-release preparation. There is no additional risk of hypoglycemia with an extended release preparation. The duration of action of second-generation sulfonylureas is as follows: glyburide, 12 to 24 hours; glipizide, 12 to 18 hours; and glimepiride, 24 hours. With sulfonylureas hypoglycemia is a frequent complication, and weight gain occurs but not as severely as with TZDs. Being sulfa drugs, they are contraindicated in patients allergic to sulfa products.

Progressive β-cell failure may require the dosage to be increased. Sulfonylureas have little effect on lipids.

New Formulations
A micronized formulation of glibenclamide (glyburide) was introduced in the U.S., which increases the rate of absorption and facilitates an earlier onset of action. A longer-acting extended-release formulation of glipizide (Glucotrol XL) is also available. A modified-release formulation of gliclazide (Diamicron MR) has been introduced. While the duration of action of gliclazide is unchanged, the new formulation uses a hydrophilic matrix to match the progressive delivery of gliclazide with the hypoglycemic profile. This improved bioavailability enables a dose reduction from 80 to 30 mg per tablet. Fixed dose combinations of glibenclamide and metformin and of glipizide and metformin are now available.

The Meglitinides

The nonsulfonylurea portion of glibenclamide, a benzamido compound termed meglitinide, was shown in the early 1980s to stimulate insulin secretion. Repaglinide was introduced in 1998 and nateglinide in 2001. These secretogogues are often termed glinides.

Repaglinide

Repaglinide interacts with a specific binding site on the SUR-1 subunit that is distinct from the glyburide sulfonylurea binding site but still causes closure of the K_{ATP} channel. Unlike sulfonylureas, repaglinide does not directly stimulate exocytosis of insulin granules. This drug targets postprandial hyperglycemia, and the insulin level returns to normal between meals, thus avoiding episodes of hypoglycemia unless the drug is taken without food. The meglitinides are completely and rapidly absorbed (repaglinide about 73%), peak plasma concentrations are achieved within an hour, and >98% of the circulatory drug is protein bound. They are rapidly metabolized by the liver and excreted mainly in the bile. When taken before meals, repaglinide, like nateglinide, produces a prompt insulin-releasing effect. They are short acting, and their insulin-releasing actions starts in 15 to 30 minutes and lasts for 4 hours (less for nateglinide). Therefore, repaglinide should be started as 0.5 mg, 30 minutes before each meal, and the time and dose should be titrated according to the size and energy content of the meals, to the maximum of 4 mg. Low dosages should always be initiated. If titrating the dose upward does not provide further benefit or a hypoglycemic attack occurs, the patient should return to the previous dose, and if a glycemic target is not met, the early use of combination therapy should be followed.

As monotherapy, repaglinide is as effective as sulfonylureas but slightly more potent than nateglinide, producing a reduction of HbA_{1c} by 1.7% and mean FPG by 62 mg/dL (3.38 mmol/L) as compared to placebo [58]. It is metabolized by cytochrome P-450 (CYP), a 3A4 system (CYP3A4 [cytochrome P450, family 3, subfamily A, polypeptide 4]) in the liver, and 90% is excreted in the bile. Repaglinide is not contraindicated in impaired renal function, but its dose should be reduced in significant liver disease. Caution should be exercised when coadministering repaglinide with gemfibrozil because there is an increased risk of hypoglycemia caused by inhibition of the metabolism of repaglinide secondary to inhibition of 3A4 by gemfibrozil. The hypoglycemia is a predominant side effect but is less marked than sulfonylureas.

The hypoglycemic effect of glinides can be potentiated by nonselective beta-blockers, salicylates, monoamine oxidase inhibitors (MAOIs), nonsteroidal antiinflammatory drugs (NSAIDs), thyroid hormones, sympathomimetic agents, and thiazide diuretics. The glinides are contraindicated in patients with type 1 diabetes. In the U.S., repaglinide and nateglinide are indicated for use as monotherapy and in combination with metformin. In Europe, the indication is the same for repaglinide, but nateglinide is only available for use in combination with metformin. Glinides are also suitable for patients who eat meals on an erratic schedule. They may also be useful for those who experience interprandial hypoglycemia.

Nateglinide
Nateglinide is a D-phenylalanine and does not contain a sulfonylurea moiety. It binds to the SUR-1 subunit of the K_{ATP} channel, but its binding characteristics are very different from those of the sulfonylureas. It is a suitable drug for reduction of postprandial glucose excursions. Nateglinide is very similar to repaglinide: it is rapidly absorbed, peaks in 2 hours, and its effects lasts for 3 hours; it metabolizes in the liver (CYP34A and CYP2C9). When given in the dose of 120 mg for 12 weeks in a patient whose glycemic control was inadequately controlled with diet and physical exercise, it resulted in a decrease of HbA_{1c} of 0.55% and a reduction of FPG of 21 mg/dL (1.11 mmol/L) [7]. If glycemic control is not achieved with sulfonylureas or metformin, the patient should not be switched to nateglinide alone. Nateglinide is not suitable for patients whose blood glucose level is >200 mg/dL (11.1 mmol/L). The hypoglycemic effects appear to be relatively mild and uncommon.

Q: How do oral combinations of antidiabetic oral agents differ in clinical efficacy?
Often the combination of two or even three agents is required especially due to the progressive nature of type 2 diabetes. In these cases, instead of replacing a drug, another drug that acts through a different mechanism should be added. This produces the additive effect of glycemic control while allowing the usage of submaximal doses. Patients presenting with an HbA_{1c} of 9% to 10% (200 to 240 mg/dL) will require more than one drug to achieve adequate glycemic control.

Metformin and Sulfonylurea
Metformin and sulfonylurea are a very popular combination as it provides additive effects on glycemic control and in reducing triglycerides and LDL cholesterol, which is important in most diabetics who are obese and have some degree of dyslipidemia. This combination

of two drugs should be given with meals with doses divided equally between breakfast and dinner. A lower dose of sulfonylurea in the combination product should be initiated to avoid hypoglycemia, particularly if the plasma glucose is less than 150 mg/dL (8.33 mmol/L). While using combination products, the side effects and combinations of both constituents should be borne in mind.

Metformin and Thiazolidinedione
Metformin and TZD are a suitable combination of two drugs. Metformin primarily inhibits hepatic gluconeogenesis and improves peripheral insulin sensitivity, whereas TZD primarily enhances insulin sensitivity in the muscle but also inhibits gluconeogenesis. Combination therapy of the two drugs reduces the HbA_{1c} by 0.8% to 1%, which can be increased to 1.3% if sulfonylurea is also added (triple therapy). A synergistic effect in lowering triglycerides and increasing HDL cholesterol is observed with the combination of metformin and TZDs.

Metformin and Repaglinide
The combination of metformin and repaglinide results in more effective glycemic control with a reduction of HbA_{1c} of 1.4% compared to 0.4% with repaglinide alone and 0.3% with metformin alone. However, the risk of hypoglycemia increases.

Metformin and Nateglinide
This combination is suitable for patients who are overweight and whose primary disturbance is postprandial hyperglycemia with HbA_{1c} <8%. The combination of the two drugs produces a reduction of the HbA_{1c} level of 1.4% and of FPG of 40 mg/dL.

Repaglinide and Thiazolidinedione
The combination of repaglinide and TZDs produces a synergistic effect that reduces the HbA_{1c} level by 1.3% after 6 months and also reduces the risk of severe hypoglycemia.

Thiazolidinedione and Insulin
Thiazolidinedione and insulin in combination is not recommended by the European guidelines.

Sulfonylurea and Thiazolidinedione
The addition of TZD to patients inadequately controlled by sulfonylureas produces synergistic effects, with a reduction of the HbA_{1c} level of 1.2% to 1.4%, slightly more than the TZD and metformin combination.

α-glucosidase Inhibitors and Sulfonylureas
Miglitol and acarbose are most effective in those patients who are on sulfonylurea and require an additional 25- to 30-mg/dL reduction in the FPG level or in those who need increased postprandial control.

Prediabetes

Q: What is the evidence that lifestyle intervention and pharmacology in prediabetes may be helpful?

On the basis of our present knowledge, there does not appear to be a single agent that can be definitely recommended for diabetes prevention. However, the following treatments have a role [88]: (1) an intensive lifestyle change aimed at modest weight loss has the strongest supportive evidence, followed by (2) bariatric surgery, (3) metformin, which has a significant effect in a specific population, (4) orlistat, acarbose, or rimonabant for obese individuals [5], and ramipril, captopril, or losartan for hypertension, (5) pravastatin in hypertension, and (6) estrogen replacement in postmenopause.

Impaired Glucose Tolerance (IGT)

The Diabetes Prevention Program (DPP) studied patients with IGT [91]. The study group was given lifestyle intervention, including advice on nutrition, prescribed physical activity for 150 minutes per week, and weight loss of 7%. The control group was given advice on healthy eating but did not receive intensive lifestyle modification support. The absolute risk of developing diabetes in the study group was 4.8% per year, compared with 11.0% per year in the control group. If this finding equates to seven people with IGT needing treatment for 1 year to prevent one new case, then the number needed to treat (NNT) per year is 7. In another arm of the DPP, metformin 850 mg twice daily in patients with IGT was compared with placebo. The incidence of diabetes in the treated group was 7.8% vs. 11.0% in the control group (NNT 20 people over 3 years). However, it is interesting that metformin was no better than placebo when used in individuals with a BMI <30, those aged >60 years, or those with fasting glucose <110 mg/dL (6.11 mmol/L). In the STOP-NIDDM trial, acarbose not only reduced the conversion to diabetes by 35% but also reduced the incidence of newly diagnosed hypertension by 34% [87]. In this study with acarbose 120 mg three times a day, diabetes developed in 17% over 3.3 years, whereas in the placebo group diabetes developed in 26%. This equates NNT to 11.5 patients treated for 3.3 years. Additionally, an appreciable reduction of overweight and triglycerides was observed. The therapeutic effects of acarbose on IGT and traits of the metabolic syndrome were associated with a significant lower incidence of major CV events. In the Finnish Diabetes Prevention Study (DPS), a comparable lifestyle modification also resulted in 3.2% of individuals in the intervention group developing diabetes, compared with 7.8% in the control group, for an NNT of five people with IGT over 5 years [90]. The results were comparable to those in the DPP.

In another study, orlistat (120 mg three times a day) when used in obese patients (BMI ≥ 30) with IGT, also resulted in an incidence of diabetes of 6.2% over 4 years vs. 9% incidence with placebo (NNT of 10 patients over 4 years) [46]. In still another study, orlistat in the dosage of 120 mg three times a day in obese (BMI ≥ 30) patients with IGT produced a 3.0% incidence of diabetes vs. 7.6% incidence with placebo (NNT 45 patients over 2 years) [93].

Obese Subjects with Normal Glucose Tolerance

There is a dearth of evidence on the success of preventing diabetes in individuals with normal glucose tolerance (NGT). However, in a meta-analysis, orlistat when used in obese patients with NGT produced an incidence of IGT of 6.6%, and none developed diabetes over 2 years, whereas those who received placebo had an incidence of 10.8% of IGT and a 1.2% incidence of diabetes over 2 years [91]. In the Swedish Obese Subjects (SOS) study (BMI ≥ 34 for men and ≥ 38 for women), those who underwent gastrointestinal surgery (as compared to nonsurgical methods) to enhance weight loss showed reductions of up to 97% in diabetes incidence at 2 and 5 years after gastric surgery, whereas the risk reduction was proportional to the magnitude of weight loss [92]. Liposuction does not appear to affect glucose metabolism.

Individuals with Hypertension

A reduction of newly diagnosed diabetes was observed in some studies with ACE inhibitors and angiotensin II receptor blockers (ARBs). The Heart Outcomes Prevention Evaluation (HOPE) investigators showed that in individuals with a history of CAD, the ACE inhibitor ramipril (10 mg daily) was associated with a decrease in the incidence of diabetes from 5.4% over 4.5 years to 3.6% in the treatment group (NNT = 56 for 4.5 years) [93]. Similarly, in the Captopril Prevention Project (CAPP), the incidence of diabetes was 15.2% over 5 years in those treated by diuretics and beta-blockers, and 13.3% in those whose hypertension was treated with captopril (NNT = 53 over 5 years) [94].

Angiotensin receptor blockers and losartan also showed promising results. In the Losartan Intervention For Endpoint (LIFE) study, the use of losartan in hypertension and left ventricular failure (LVF) reduced the incidence of diabetes from 1.75% per year in those using beta-blockers (atenolol) to 1.30% (NNT =222 per year) [95]. However, in the Diabetes REduction Approaches with ramipril and rosiglitazone Medication (DREAM) study, ramipril did not show a reduction in the primary end point or in its separate components, meaning that ACE inhibitors should no longer be considered a protective diabetic preventive strategy [96].

Hyperlipidemia

In the WOSCOP study, the use of pravastatin 40 mg daily reduced the risk of developing diabetes from 2.8% in those treated with placebo to 1.9% (NNT = 111 for 5.5 years) [97].

Postmenopausal Women

Hormone replacement therapy (HRT) appears to confer beneficial effects. However, when prescribed for the prevention of diabetes, the patients' needs should be balanced against the other risks of these drugs. The Estrogen/Progesterone Replacement Study showed that in postmenopausal women HRT (0.62 mg of conjugated estrogens plus 2.5 mg of medroxyprogesterone daily) was associated with a 6% incidence over 4.1 years as compared to 10% in women treated with placebo (30 patients needed to treat for 4.1 years to prevent one case) [98].

Hypertension

Q: What are the indications for lifestyle modification and pharmacotherapy in hypertension?

The seventh report of the JNC classifies blood pressure (BP) as follows: (1) normal, systolic <120 mm Hg and diastolic <80 mm Hg; (2) prehypertension, systolic 120 to 139 mm Hg or diastolic 80 to 89 mm Hg; (3) hypertension: stage I, systolic 140 to 159 mm Hg or diastolic 90 to 99 mm Hg; stage II, systolic 160 to 179 mm Hg or diastolic 100 to 109 mm Hg; stage III, systolic ≥180 mm Hg or diastolic ≥110 mm Hg.

The BP goal is <135/<85 mm Hg, but in the presence of diabetes or chronic kidney disease, it is <130/85 mm Hg. The vast majority of individuals with the metabolic syndrome fall into the categories of prehypertension or stage I hypertension [99]. In those aged >50 years, a systolic blood pressure of >140 is a more important risk factor than the diastolic blood pressure. Beginning at 115/77 mm Hg, the CVD risk doubles for each increment of

20/10 mm Hg; those who are normotensive at the age of 55 years, will have a 90% lifetime risk of developing hypertension. The relationship between BP and the rise of CVD events is continuous, consistent, and independent of other risk factors. The higher the BP, the greater the chance of heart attack, heart failure, stroke, and kidney disease. Hypertension should be treated according to the seventh report of the JNC [100].

In the treatment of hypertension, lifestyle measures should always precede or accompany the pharmacological therapy. Prehypertensive subjects require health promotion and lifestyle modification to prevent the progressive rise in BP or in the incidence of CVD. This includes cessation of smoking, increased physical activity, reduction of weight (if overweight), and consumption of a healthy diet (including increased consumption of fruits and vegetables, low-fat dairy products, and the DASH diet, which was discussed earlier in this chapter) [27]. In some individuals, a 1600-mg sodium DASH eating plan has a blood pressure effect similar to that of single drug therapy. Supplementation of the diet with 60 to 120 mmol of potassium daily reduces the systolic and diastolic blood pressure by 4.4 and 2.5 mm Hg, respectively, in hypertension and by 1.8 and 1.0 mm Hg, respectively, in normotensive patients. Weight reduction is associated with reduction of blood pressure. The loss of 4 kg in body weight is associated with a mean decrease in blood pressure of 1 mm Hg. Salt restriction can independently reduce blood pressure and is additive with weight loss. Moderate restriction of salt, to no more than 100 mmol (2.4 g of sodium) per day can reduce the systolic blood pressure by 5 mm Hg and the diastolic pressure by 2 to 3 mm Hg [100]. Physical activity, involving 30 to 45 minutes of brisk walking, is associated with lowering of the blood pressure, as is smoking cessation and reduction of alcohol intake. Advice on weight reduction can be obtained at www.nhlbi.nih.gov. and www.americanheart.org.

Drug therapy is indicated in those whose blood pressure cannot be controlled with lifestyle measures, to prevent MI, stroke, and kidney disease. The four classes of drugs most commonly used either as monotherapy or in combination are beta-blockers (BBs), calcium channel blockers (CCBs), ACE inhibitors/angiotensin II blockers (ARBs), and diuretics. However, due to recent evidence of the adverse effects of BB on glucose tolerance, CCB, ACE/ARB, and diuretics are preferred. Other drugs such as α-blockers, methyldopa, and clonidine may have a role as an adjunctive therapy where blood pressure is difficult to control or there is a compelling indication [99].

No hypertensive agent has been identified as being preferable for individuals with the metabolic syndrome. Diuretics or BBs in high doses can worsen insulin resistance and atherogenic dyslipidemia. For uncomplicated hypertension, thiazide diuretics should be prescribed [99]. For high-risk conditions that are compelling indications, alternative antihypertensives should be prescribed.

Most patients require two, three, or even four antihypertensives to achieve target BP, particularly when associated with diabetes or renal disease. Besides lowering the blood pressure, certain antihypertensive agents may have a pleiotropic effect on the physiology of the metabolic syndrome. For thiazide diuretics, the doses should be kept relatively low. At the present time, the majority of clinical trials indicate that most risk reduction associated with antihypertensives is the result of the blood pressure lowering alone. However, there is substantial evidence that ACE inhibitors and ARBs may lower the risk of diabetes. In individuals with IFG and IGT, diuretics increase the likelihood of developing diabetes, although they reduce CV events. The ACE inhibitors have advantages in individuals with CV disease, nephropathy, and retinopathy; they have been shown to reduce complication rates in the UKPDS study [101].

Angiotensin-Converting Enzyme Inhibitors/Angiotensin II Blockers

Q: What are the advantages of ACE inhibitors and ARBs in the treatment of the metabolic syndrome and CVD prevention?
The angiotensin-converting enzyme (ACE) converts inactive angiotensin I to active angiotensin II. The ACE inhibitors are effective in lowering blood pressure, are metabolically neutral, have a good side-effect profile, reverse left ventricular hypertrophy, and are the drug of choice in CHF. The ACE inhibitors and ARBs have been shown to improve insulin resistance in several studies but not in all. Inhibition of the rennin-angiotensin system with ACE inhibitors/ARBs reduces the risk of developing diabetes and reduces albumin loss in diabetic patients with microalbuminuria.

While choosing an antihypertensive drug to initiate the treatment, the medical history (including age, gender, ethnicity, family history, and presence of diabetes) and compelling indications should be taken into account. Some drugs are more beneficial in certain groups. Some clinicians prefer ACE inhibitors as first-line therapy for hypertension in the metabolic syndrome especially when the patient also has type 2 diabetes or chronic kidney disease. The ARBs are indicated in those who are unable to tolerate ACE inhibitors, and some clinicians go as far as using ARBs as a preferred choice over ACE inhibitors when diabetes is present.

At higher doses ACE inhibitors and ARBs are shown to be reno- and cardioprotective. They decrease the elevated systemic vascular resistance, reduce sympathetic tone, and increase perfusion of heart and kidneys. In the HOPE study of 5720 high-risk patients with CVD (aged over 55 years, duration of study 4.5 years), the cardiovascular protective effect was greater than the effects of blood pressure lowering. The intervention and relative risk for diabetes of ramipril vs. placebo was 35% (p <.005) [102] (Table 6.4).

The Capp study of 10,413 patients with hypertension (ages 25 to 66 years, duration of study 6.1 years) compared ACE inhibitor and captopril with a BB or thiazide. In 600 diabetic patients there was no difference in blood pressure, but the ACE inhibitor showed significant reduction in MI of 34% and cardiac events of 67% (intervention and relative risk for diabetes of captopril vs. BB/thiazide was 14%, p <.005) [94].

Side effects: Persistent cough is often the reason for discontinuation of therapy; the ARBs are alternative drugs in these patients.

TABLE 6.4. The doses of ACE inhibitors and ARBs in hypertension (refer to the prescribing information relevant to your national formulary and guidelines)

	Daily dose range (mg/d)	Frequency	Initial dose (mg)
ACE inhibitors			
Benazepril	10–40	1	5
Captopril	25–100	2	12.5–25
Enalapril	5–40	1–2	2.5–5
Fonisopril	10–40	1	5–10
Lisinopril	10–40	1	2.5–5
Moexipril	7.5–30	1	7.5
Perindopril	4–8	1	1–2
Quinapril	10–80	1	2.5–5
Ramipril	2.5–20	1	1.25–2.5
Trandolapril	1–4	1	0.5
ARBs			
Candesartan	8–32	1	4–8
Eprosartan	400–800	1–2	300–400
Irbesartan	150–300	1	75–150
Losartan	25–100	1–2	50
Olmesartan	20–40	1	10
Telmisartan	20–80	1	20
Valsartan	80–300	1–2	40

First-dose hypotension is rare but reported; therefore, therapy should be initiated at the lowest dose and titrated to the appropriate dose over several weeks. Discontinuation of diuretics for a day before and just after starting an ACE inhibitor may reduce the hypotensive effect. These drugs may also cause renal impairment and angioneurotic edema; therefore, they are contraindicated in patients known to be hypersensitive to these symptoms, or those known or suspected to have renovascular disease or in cases of renal artery stenosis. Serum creatinine, therefore, should be checked before starting therapy, and checked again 7 to 10 days after starting therapy and after each dose increment. Other side effects include altered liver function tests, cholestatic jaundice, hepatitis, and blood disorders.

Angiotensin II Receptor Blockers

The ARBs, like the ACE inhibitors, also inhibit the rennin-angiotensin system but through a direct blocking effect of the angiotensin II (AT-II) receptor. Almost all recognized effects of AT-II are mediated by the AT-I receptors, which are blocked by AT-I receptor antagonist drugs. These drugs have both a cardiac and renal protective effect and are also useful in heart failure. The renal protective effect is beyond and possibly unrelated to the lowering of BP. The ARBs not only are antihypertensive but also have the following cardioprotective effects: (1) improve endothelial function; (2) improve left ventricular hypertrophy (LVH) and arterial mass better than other antihypertensives; and (3) reduce rates of death, MI, stroke, cardiac arrest, and revascularization procedures. The ACE inhibitors protect against oxidative stress and prevent glycosylation of proteins, which may provide CV benefit.

Most of the work with type 1 diabetes has been with ACE inhibitors, whereas in patients with type 2 diabetes, hypertension and microalbuminuria have resulted using ARBs, which have been shown to prevent and retard progression from incipient (microalbuminuria) to overt (macroproteinuria) nephropathy and slow the progression of established diabetic renal disease. The results of some studies support the current view that inhibition of the rennin-angiotensin system, whether by ACE inhibitors or ARBs confer renal and cardioprotection.

Insulin resistance results in overactivity of rennin-angiotensin-aldosterone system (RAAS), leading to hypertrophy and stiffening of smooth muscles in the arterial wall and left ventricle. The ACE inhibitors and ARBs have a proven efficacy for improving the outcome in insulin-resistant conditions, such as hypertension, CHD, and CHF, and they are the most effective antihypertensive agents for improving the smooth muscle hypertrophy commonly seen in these conditions. Large numbers of trials suggest that there is a reduction in the development of new-onset diabetic cases with the antihypertensive agents. These trials predominantly used ACE inhibitors and ARBs, which produced consistent results of reduction in the risk of new diabetes ranging from 4% to 87%. In the presence of insulin resistance, the cardiovascular system is sensitized to the adverse trophic effects of RAAS, as suggested by the frequent presence of diffuse arterial disease and LVH in diabetic patients, even though their BP and lipids are normal. High insulin levels stimulate the angiotensin I receptor, which activates the RAAS, and also increases cardiac sympathetic nervous system function. The HOPE study and Microalbuminuria Cardiovascular and Renal Outcomes (MICRO-HOPE) substudy showed a reduction of CV mortality of up to 40% with ramipril [95].

Thus, in a patient with conditions associated with insulin resistance, such as the metabolic syndrome, hypertension, IFG, family history of diabetes, obesity, CHF, or other risks for the development of type 2 diabetes, the use of ACE inhibitors or ARBs should be considered. The ARBs are recommended by the ADA as the first-line treatment for diabetics with diabetic nephropathy. In the Losartan Intervention FOR Endpoint reduction (LIFE) study, ARBs reduced the rate of CV events. The primary composite end point of CV mortality, fatal/nonfatal stroke, fatal/nonfatal MI was reduced by almost 15% ($p < .0009$) in the ARB group, compared with the beta-blocker group. The result is largely attributable to a risk reduction in stroke (intervention and relative risk for diabetes of losartan vs. atenolol was 25%, $p < .0005$) [95].

Irbesartan Nephropathy Diabetic Trial (IDNT), which included 1700 hypertensive type 2 diabetic patients and lasted for a duration of 3 years, compared the effects of irbesartan with placebo and the CCB amlodipine in patients with normal or raised creatinine and with significant proteinuria. The primary outcome was the time to the composite end point of doubling of baseline creatinine level, end-stage renal disease, and death. For the primary end point, the irbesartan group showed a relative risk reduction of 20% compared to placebo ($p = .02$) and 23% compared to amlodipine ($p = .006$) [103]. The Reduction of Endpoints in NIDDM with the Angiotensin II antagonist Losartan (RENNAL) study compared the ARB losartan with placebo in hypertensive type 2 diabetic patients with proteinuria. The relative risk reduction for the primary composite end point (similar to that in IDNT) was 16% compared to the control group ($p = .02$) [104].

Also, there is some evidence that these two agents (ACE inhibitors and ARBs) have an additive effect, not only in lowering BP even further but also in correcting renal protein leakage [105].

β-Adrenoceptor Blockers Agents

Q: Should beta-blockers no longer be the first choice in the metabolic syndrome?

Beta-blockers (β-adrenoceptor blocking agents) are relatively inexpensive and effective in lowering blood pressure, with evidence of CV protection, particularly after an MI. However, they have several adverse effects, including metabolic disturbances. The studies show that BB precipitates the onset of diabetes. The use of atenolol in the UKPDS 1998 study was associated with significant higher levels of HBA_{1c} and weight gain compared with captopril. Beta-blockers, even β_1-selective drugs, also increase triglycerides, lower HDL cholesterol, and worsen insulin sensitivity. There are consistent data from prospective studies that show that they precipitate the onset of diabetes [105]. Therefore, BBs do not appear to be an appropriate first choice of antihypertensive agent unless there are indications for doing so, such as in post-MI cases.

Previously, the British Hypertensive Society and ATP-III had formulated an "AB/CD" algorithm for the stepwise treatment of hypertension. Each letter of the algorithm refers to a different BP-lowering class of drugs. The "ACD" algorithm (Fig. 6.1) is a

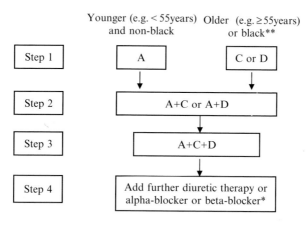

FIGURE 6.1. Revised National Institute of Clinical Excellence (NICE)/ British Hypertensive Society (BHS) treatment algorithm for newly diagnosed hypertension® NICE/BHS guidelines, 2006. A, angiotensin-converting enzyme (ACE) inhibitor or angiotensin-II antagonist; C, calcium-channel blocker; D, diuretic (thiazides-type); *, consider seeking specialist advice; **, black patients are those of African or Caribbean descent, not mixed race, Asians, or Chinese.

replacement of the previously used "AB/CD," (where B stood for beta-blockers), in light of the recently published BP-lowering arm of the Anglo-Scandinavian Cardiac Outcomes Trial (ASCOT-BPLA) [105], for newly diagnosed hypertension by the National Institute of Clinical Excellence (NICE)/British Hypertensive Society (BHS) (www.nice.UK/CG034). US still follows AB/CD algorithm. The ASCOT-BPLA study was designed to compare the effects of the combination of BB and thiazides (bendroflumethiazide) vs. CCB (amlodipine) and ACE inhibitor (perindopril), on the primary prevention of CV disease in subjects with hypertension with at least three other CV risk factors. A total of 26% of participants in each treatment group had type 2 diabetes. The trial was prematurely stopped because of the higher prevalence of CV events and death in the BB and thiazides arm. Additionally, there was a statistically significant 30% increase in new-onset diabetes as compared to the CCB group ($p < .001$). As a result of new guidelines, BBs are no longer recommended as a routine therapy for newly diagnosed hypertensive patient [105].

The ACE inhibitors (A) or beta-blockers (B) are generally more effective as initial therapy in younger white patients than are CCBs (C) or diuretics (D). However, CCBs or diuretics are a more effective initial therapy for older white individuals or black people of any age. However, beta-blockers can be considered for (1) younger individuals, particularly for women of childbearing potential; (2) patients with evidence of increased sympathetic drive, and (3) individuals with intolerance of or contraindication to ACE inhibitors and ARBs. If an individual is taking a beta-blocker and needs a second drug, a CCB should be added rather than thiazide-type diuretic to reduce the patient's risk of developing diabetes. The BHS recommends that if a patient's blood pressure is well controlled by a regimen that includes a BB, then consider long-term management at the patient's routine review. There is no need to replace the BB in this case. The BB should not usually be withdrawn if a patient has a compelling indication for being treated with one, such as symptomatic angina or a previous MI.

Calcium channel blockers are inexpensive, effective in reducing blood pressure, and have peripheral vasodilating properties. They also have additional benefits of antianginal, antiarrhythmic, and cardioprotective effects. They are metabolically neutral, and there is evidence that they improve the coronary blood flow and the left ventricular hypertrophy.

Thiazides are inexpensive and have been used for a long time. They have a well-known safety profile, but lately their propensity to deteriorate the glucose metabolism has caused concern.

However, they provide cardioprotection, with a reduction in the incidence of stroke, heart failure, and the risk of CV disease. They can provoke hypokalemia and erectile dysfunction. Most clinicians are of the opinion that the potential benefit of low-dose diuretics in combination with other antihypertensive agents outweighs their risk.

Peripheral Vascular Disease

Q: What is the association of peripheral vascular disease and the metabolic syndrome?
Peripheral vascular disease (PVD) is a common condition, with a prevalence of 4.5% among people aged 55 to 74 years. Risk factors include advanced age, male sex, high cholesterol, smoking, type 2 diabetes, and hypertension. Cigarette smoking is the strongest risk factor. Most individuals are asymptomatic and do not develop classic claudication symptoms. Claudicants typically present with pain in a muscle group, usually the calf muscle on walking a certain distance. Disease of the iliac arteries produces hip, buttock, and thigh claudication, whereas disease in the femoral and popliteal arteries produces calf claudication. The diagnosis is established by measuring the ankle brachial pressure index, which is found to be <0.9 (normal is >1). Some of the components of the metabolic syndrome also increase the likelihood and nature of PVD. These include procoagulant factors, diabetes, dyslipidemia, and hypertension. Diabetes, raised LDL cholesterol, and high blood pressure are common associations. The Edinburgh Artery Study reported a quarter of study population had the metabolic syndrome [106]. In that study the ATP-III definition of the metabolic syndrome was used, but waist circumference was replaced by BMI (cutoff for men 28.8 and for women 26.7). Diabetes is an important risk factor for peripheral arterial disease (PAD) and atherosclerotic coronary disease. However, in diabetes, besides atherosclerosis, other factors such as neuropathy, microangiopathy, and susceptibility to infection play a role in producing the classic ischemic lower limb, often seen in the past. There is a greater association between PAD and impaired glucose tolerance or diabetes.

Both elevated triglycerides and high LDL cholesterol are risk factors for PVD (go to www.hena.radcliffe-oxford.com/PADframe.html for further information). With blood pressure, PAD has a varying relationship. However, systolic blood pressure appears to play some role. Hemostatic (e.g., elevated level of fibrinogen and fibrin D-dimer) and inflammatory markers (e.g., CRP) may play a role in the development of PAD. In patients with claudication, a high level of D-dimer was an important predictor of CV events. The National Health and Nutrition Examination Survey (NHANES) found that those in the highest quartile of fibrinogen and CRP had an odds ratio for PAD of 2.7 and 2.3, respectively, compared with those in the lowest quartile [107]. Albuminuria, a marker of renal dysfunction, was observed to be positively related to PAD to the same severity as smoking in a study of American Indians with a high prevalence of diabetes. However, no definite positive correlation is observed with excessive alcohol intake and lack of exercise, though exercise improves symptoms of claudication. In the treatment of PVD, the following have a role: (1) smoking cessation, (2) lipid-lowering therapy, (3) antihypertensive treatment, (4) diabetes control, (5) antiplatelet therapy, (6) cilostazol, and (7) supervised walking exercise.

References

1. Isomaa B, Almgren P, Tuomi T, et al. Cardiovascular morbidity and mortality associated with the metabolic syndrome. Diabetes Care 2001;24:683–689.
2. Wilson PW. Estimating CVD risk and the metabolic syndrome: Framingham view. Endocrinol Metab Clin North Am 2004;33:467–481.
3. Eckel RH, Grundy SM, Zimmet P. The metabolic syndrome. Lancet 2005;365:9468–9415.
4. Grundy SM. Metabolic syndrome: connecting and reconciling CV and diabetes world. J Am Coll Cardiol 2006;47:1093–1100.
5. Lemieux I, Pascot A, Couillard C, et al. Hypertriglyceridemic waist: a marker of the atherogenic metabolic triad. Circulation 2000;102:179–184.
6. Assman G, Cullen P, Schulte H, et al. Simple scoring scheme for calculating the risk of acute coronary events based on the 10-year follow-up of the PROCAM Study. Circulation 2002;105:310–315.
7. Kahn R, Buse J, Ferrannini E, et al. The metabolic syndrome: time for a clinical appraisal. Diabetes Care 2005;28:2289–2304.
8. Pyora K, Ballantyne CM, Gumbiner B, et al. Reduction of CV events by simvastatin in nondiabetic CHD patients with or without the metabolic syndrome. Diabetes Care 2004;27:1735–1740.
9. GISSI Prevenzione Investigators. Dietary supplementation with n-3 polyunsaturated fatty acids and vitamin E after myocardial infarction. Lancet 1999;354:447–455.
10. Zarraga I, Ignatius GE, Schwarz E. Impact of dietary patterns and intervention on cardiovascular health. Circulation 2006;114:961–973.
11. Grundy SM, Cleeman JI, Daniels SR, et al. Diagnosis and management of the metabolic syndrome (AHA/NHLBI). Circulation 2005;112:2735–2752.
12. Hu FB, Stampfer MJ, Manson JE, et al. Dietary fat intake and the risk of CHD in women. N Engl J Med 1997;337:1491–1499.

13. Vessby B, Unsitupa M, Hermansen K, et al. Substituting dietary saturated for monosaturated fat impairs insulin sensitivity in healthy men and women. Diabetologia 2001;44:312–319.
14. de Lorgeril M, Salen P, Bontemps L, et al. Mediterranean diet, traditional risk factors and the rate of CV complications after myocardial infarction. Circulation 1999;99:779.
15. Sevak L, McKeigne PM, Mermot MG. Relation of hyperinsulinaemia in dietary intake in South Asians and European man. Am J Clin Nutr 1994;59:1069–1074.
16. Brady LM, Williams CM, Lovegrove JA. Dietary PUFA and the metabolic syndrome in Indian Asians living in the UK. Proc Nutr Soc 2004;63:115–125.
17. Jenkins DJ, Kendall CW, Marchie A, et al. Effects of dietary portfolio of cholesterol-lowering foods vs lovastatin on serum lipids and CRP. JAMA 2003;290:502–510.
18. Klien S, Burke LE, Bray GA, et al. Clinical implications of obesity with specific focus on CVD. Circulation 2004;110:2952–2967.
19. Jarvi AE, Darlstrom BE, Granfeldt YE et al. Improved glycaemic control and lipid profile and normalized fibrinolytic activity on a low-glycaemic index diet in type 2 diabetes patient. Diabetes Care 1999;22:10–18.
20. Giugliano D, Ceriello A, Epsosito K. The effects of diet on inflammation. J Am Coll Cardiol 2006;48:677–685.
21. The KUOPIO Ischemic Disease Risk Factors (KIHD) Study. J Nutr 2003;133:199–204.
22. Ajani UA, Ford ES, Mokdad AL. Dietary fiber and CRP: finding from NHANES data. J Nutr 2004;134:1181–1185.
23. McAuley RA, Williams SM, Mann JI, et al. Intensive lifestyle changes are necessary to improve insulin sensitivity: a randomized controlled trial. Diabetes Care 2002;25:445–452.
24. McAuley KA, Hopkins CM, Smith KJ, et al. Composition of high-fat and high-protein diets with a high-carbohydrate diet in insulin-resistant obese women. Diabetologia 2005;48:8–16.
25. Esposito K, Marfella R, Ciotola M, et al. Effects of Mediterranean-style diet on endothelial dysfunction and markers of vascular inflammation in the metabolic syndrome: a randomized trial. JAMA 2004;292:1440–1446.
26. Burr MC, Felicity AM, Gilbert JF, et al. Effects of changes in fat, fish and fiber intakes on death and myocardial infarction. Lancet 1989;2:757–761.
27. Azadbakht L, Mirmiran P, Esmaillzadeh A, et al. Beneficial effects and DASH: eating plan on features of metabolic syndrome. Diabetes Care 2005;28:2823–2831.
28. Rimm ED, Klatsky A, Grobbee D, et al. Review of moderate alcohol consumption and reduced risk of CHD: is the effect due to beer, wine or spirit. BMJ 1996;312:731–736.
29. Mukamal KJ, Maclure M, Miller E, et al. Binge drinking and mortality after acute myocardial infarction. Circulation 2005;112:3839–3845.

30. Mukamal KJ, Jensen MK, Grouback M, et al. Drinking frequency mediating biomarkers, and risk of myocardial infarction in women and men. Circulation 2005;112:1406–1413.

31. Yoon YS, Oh SW, Baik HW, et al. Alcohol consumption and the metabolic syndrome in Korean (NHANES). Am J Clin Nutr 2004;80(1):217–224.

32. Rusell M, De Faire U, Hellenius ML. Low prevalence of metabolic syndrome in wine drinkers. Eur J Clin Nutr 2003;57(2):227–234.

33. Stanner S. Cardiovascular Disease: Diet, Nutrition and Emerging Risk Factors. British Nutrition Foundation. London: Blackwell, 2005.

34. Thompson P, Buchner D, Pina IL, et al. Exercise and physical activity in the prevention and treatment of atherosclerotic CVD (AHA Scientific Statement). Circulation 2003;107:3109–3116.

35. Laaksonen D, Lakka H, Salonen J, et al. LTPA and cardiovascular and respiratory fitness predict the development of metabolic syndrome. Diabetes Care 2002;25:1612–1618.

36. Leon AS, Sanchez O. Meta analysis of the effects of aerobic exercise training on blood lipids. Circulation 2001;104:11414–11415.

37. Klein BE, Klein R, Lee KE. Components of metabolic syndrome and risk of CVD and diabetes in Beaver Dam. Diabetes Care 2002;25:1790–1794.

38. Wilson PWF, Grundy SM. The metabolic syndrome. Circulation 2003;108:1422–1430.

39. Haffner SM, Despres J-P, Dalkau B, et al. Waist circumference and BMI are both independently associated with CVD. J Am Coll Cardiol 2006;47(suppl A):358A.

40. Watkins LL, Sherwood A, Feinglos M, et al. Effects of exercise and weight loss on cardiac risk factors associated with syndrome X. Arch Intern Med 2003;163:1889–1895.

41. Ebbeling CB, Leidig MM, Sinclair KB, et al. A reduced-glycemic load diet in the treatment of adolescent obesity. Arch Pediatr Adolesc Med 2003;157:773–779.

42. Haddock CK, Poston NS, Dill PL, et al. Pharmacotherapy for obesity. Int J Obes Relat Metab Disord 2002;26:262–244.

43. Arterburn DE, Crane PK, Veenstra DL, et al. The efficacy and safety of sibutramine for weight loss. Arch Intern Med 2004;164:994–1003.

44. Apfelbaun M, Vague P, Ziegler O, et al. Long-term maintenance of weight loss after a very low calorie diet. Am J Med 1999;106:179–184.

45. Padwal R, Li SK, Laud DC, et al. Long-term pharmacotherapy for overweight and obesity. Int J Obes 2003;27:1437–1446.

46. Torgerson JS, Hauptmann J, Boldrin MN et al. Xanical in the Prevention of Diabetes in Obese Subjects (XENDOS) study. Diabetes Care 2004;27:155–161.

47. Pi-Sunyer FX, Aronne LJ, Heshmati HM, et al. The RIO-North American Study; effects of rimonabant. JAMA 2006;295:761–775.

48. Gadde KM, Allison DB. Cannabinoid-1 receptor antagonist, rimonabant, for management of obesity and related risks. Circulation 2006;114:974–984.

49. Kolovou GD, Anagnostopoulou KK, Cokkinos DV. Pathophysiology of dyslipidemia in the metabolic syndrome. Postgrad Med J 2005; 81:358–366.

50. Knopp RH, Walden CE, Retzlaff BM, et al. Long-term cholesterol-lowering effects of 4 fat-restricted diets in hypercholesterolemia and combined hyperlipidemic men. JAMA 1997;278:1509–1515.

51. NCEP 3rd Report. Expert Panel on Detection, Evaluation, and Treatment of High Blood Cholesterol. Circulation 2002;106:3343–3321.

52. Meyers CD, Kashyap ML. Management of the metabolic syndrome-nicotinic acid. Endocrinol Metab Clin North Am 2004;33(3):557–575.

53. Brown BG, Zhao XQ, Chait A, et al. Simvastatin and niacin, antioxidant vitamin, or the combination for the prevention of coronary disease. N Engl J Med 2001;345:1583–1592.

54. Byrne CD, Wild SH. The Metabolism Syndrome. New York: John Wiley & Sons, 2005.

55. Staels B, Dallongeville J, Auwerx J, et al. Mechanism of action of fibrates on lipid and lipoprotein metabolism. Circulation 1998;98(19): 2088–2093.

56. Steiner G. The use of fibrates and of statin in preventing atherosclerosis in diabetes. Curr Opin Lipidol 2001;12(6):611–617.

57. Frick MH, Elo O, Haap K, et al. The Helsinki Heart Study. Primary prevention trial with gemfibrozil in middle-aged men with dyslipidemia. N Engl J Med 1987;317(20):1237–1245.

58. Rubins HB, Robins SJ, Collin SD et al. Gemfibrozil for secondary prevention of CHD in men with low levels of HDL-C. N Engl J Med 1999;341:410–418.

59. Otvos JD, Collins D, Freedman S, et al. LDL- and HDL particle subclasses predict coronary events and are favorably changed by gemfibrozil therapy in the VA-HIT. Circulation 2006;113:1156–1163.

60. Vakkilainen J, Steiner G, Ansquer JC. Relationship between LDL particle size, plasma lipoproteins, and progression of coronary artery disease. Circulation 2003;107(13):1733–1737.

61. Martin G, Duez H, Blangnart C, et al. Statin-induced inhibition of the Rho-signaling pathway activates PPARα and induces HDL ApoA-I. J Clin Invest 2001;107:1423–1432.

62. Schonbeck U, Libby P. Inflammation and HMG-CoA reductase inhibitors. Circulation 2004;109(suppl II):18–28.

63. Masou RD, Walter M, Jacob F. Effects of HMG-CoA reductase inhibitors on endothelial function. Circulation 2004;109(suppl II):34–41.

64. Wassmann S, Lauf U, Muller K et al. Cellular antioxidant effects of atorvastatin in vitro and in vivo. Arterioscler Thromb Vasc Biol 2002;22:300–305.

65. PedersenTR, Faergeman O, kastelein JJ, et al. High-dose atorvastatin vs. usual-dose simvastatin for secondary prevention after myocardial infarction. JAMA 2005;294:2437–2445.

66. Freeman DJ, Morrie J, Sattar N, et al. Pravastatin and the development of diabetes mellitus, evidence for a protective treatment effect in the WOSCOP Study. Circulation 2003;103:357–362.

67. Colhoun HM, Betteridge DJ, Durrington P, et al. Primary prevention of CVD with atorvastatin in type 2 diabetes in the CARDS. Lancet 2004;364:685–696.

68. Albert MA, Daniel E, Rifai R. The pravastatin inflammation/CRP evaluation. JAMA 2001;286(1):64–70.

69. Costa A, Casamitjana R, Casals E, et al. Effects of atorvastatin on glucose homoeostasis, postprandial triglyceride response and CRP in subjects with impaired fasting glucose. Diabet Med 2003; 20(9): 743–745.

70. UKPDS. Effective intensive blood glucose control with metformin on complications in overweight patients with type 2 diabetes. Lancet 1998;352:854–865.

71. Khan CR, Weir GC, King GL. Joslin's Diabetes Mellitus. Philadelphia: Lippincott Williams & Wilkins, 2005.

72. Yang W-S, Jeng C-Y, Wu J-J, et al. Synthetic PPAR-γ agonists, rosiglitazone, increase plasma level of adiponectin in type 2 diabetes patient. Diabetes Care 2002;25:376–380.

73. Dormandy JA, Charbonnel B, Eckland DJ et al. PROspective pioglitAzone Clinical Trial in macro Vascular Events. Lancet 2005;366:1279–1289.

74. Freemantle N. How well does the evidence on pioglitazone back up researchers' claims for a reduction in macrovascular events. BMJ 2005;331:836–838.

75. Goldberg RB, Kendall DM, Deeg M, et al. A comparison of lipid and glycaemic effect of pioglitazone and rosiglitazone in patients with type 2 diabetes and dyslipidemia. Diabetes Care 2005; 28:1547–1554.

76. Steals B. PPAR-γ and atherosclerosis. Curr Med Res Opin 2005; 2(suppl 1):S13–S20.

77. Sidhu JS, Cowan D, Kaski JC. Effects of rosiglitazone on endothelial function in men with CAD without diabetes. Am J Cardiol 2004;94:151–156.

78. Delerive P, Martin-Nazard F, Chinetti G, et al. PPAR activators inhibit thrombin-induced ET-1 production in human vascular endothelial cells by inhibiting the activator protein signaling pathway. Circ Res 1999;85:394–402.

79. Cho D-H, Chor YJ, Jo SA, et al. NO production and regulation of endothelial NO synthase phosphorylation by prolonged treatment with troglitazone. J Biol Chem 2004;279:2499–2506.

80. Wang P, Anderson PO, Chen S, et al. Inhibition of the transcription factors, A P-1, NF-kappa-B in CD4 T cells by PPAR-γ ligands. Int. Immunopharmacology 2001;1:802–803.

81. Chinetti G, Fruchart J-C, Staels B. PPAR-γ: nuclear receptors at the crossroads between lipid metabolism and inflammation. Inflamm Res 2000;49:497–505.

82. Liang C-P, Han S, Okamoto H, et al. Increased CD36 protein as response to defective insulin signaling in macrophages. J Clin Invest 2004;133:764–773.

83. Goetze S, Xi XP, Kawanto H, et al. PPARγ–ligands inhibit migration mediated by multiple chemoattractant in vascular smooth muscle cells. J Cardiovasc Pharmacol 1999;33:798–806.
84. Rampamelli S, Rinaldi T, Perriello G, et al. Effects of pioglitazone on coagulation and thrombosis in comparison in patient with type 2 diabetes. 64th Sci Session ADA, Orlando, June 4–8, 2004.
85. Lebovitz HE. α-Glucosidase inhibitors as agents in the treatment of diabetes. Diabetes Rev 1998;6:132–145.
86. Hanefield M, Cagaty M, Petrowitch T, et al. Acarbose reduces the risk of myocardial infarction in type 2 diabetic patients. Eur Heart J 2004;25(1):10–16.
87. Chiasson Jl, Josse RG, Gomis R, et al. Acarbose for the prevention of type 2 diabetes: STOP-NIDDM trial. Lancet 2002;3591:2072–2077.
88. Curtis J, Wilson C. Preventing type 2 diabetes mellitus. J Am Board Fam Pract 2005;18:37–43.
89. Knowler WC, Barrett-Connor E, Fowler SE, et al. Reduction in the incidence of type 2 diabetes with lifestyle intervention or metformin (DPP). N Engl J Med 2002;346:393–403.
90. Tuomilehto J, Lindstrom J, Eriksson JG, et al. Prevention of type 2 diabetes mellitus by changes in lifestyle among subjects with impaired glucose tolerance. N Engl J Med 2001;344:1343–1350.
91. Heymsfield SB, Segal KR, Hauptman J, et al. Effects of weight loss with orlistat on glucose tolerance and progression of type 2 diabetes in obese adults. Arch Intern Med 2000;160:1321–1326.
92. Sjostrom CD, Lissner L, Wedel H, et al. Reduction in the incidence of diabetes, hypertension and lipid disturbances after intentional weight loss induced by bariatric surgery. Obes Res 1999;7:477–484.
93. Yusuf S, Gerstein H, Hoogwerf B, et al. Ramipril and the development of diabetes. JAMA 2001;286:1882–1885.
94. CAPP study. Effect of angiotensin II blockers compared with conventional therapy on CV morbidity and mortality in hypertension. Lancet 1999;353:611–616.
95. Lindholm LH, Ibsen H, Borch-Johnsen K, et al. Risk of new onset diabetes in the LIFE study. J Hypertension 2002;20:1879–1886.
96. DREAM investigators. Effects of ramipril on the incidence of diabetes. N Engl J Med 2006;355:1551–1562.
97. Freeman DJ, Norie J, Sattar N, et al. Pravastatin and the development of diabetes mellitus. Evidence for a protective treatment effect in WOSCOPS. Circulation 2001;103:351–362.
98. Kanaya AM, Herrington D, Vittinghoff E, et al. Glycemic effects of postmenopausal hormone therapy. Ann Intern Med 2003;139:1–9.
99. Chobanian AV, Bakris GL, Black HR, et al. JNC report. Hypertension 2003;42:1204–1252.
100. Cutler JA, Follmann D, Allender PS. Randomized trials of sodium restriction. Am J Clin Nutr 1997;65(suppl 2):643S–651S.
101. Stearne MR, Palmer SL, Hammersley MS, et al. UKPDS. Tight blood pressure control and risk of macro vascular and microvascular complications in type 2 diabetes. Br Med J 1998;317:703–713.

102. Effects of ramipril on CV and microvascular outcomes in people with diabetes mellitus. Lancet 2000;355:252–259.
103. Lewis EJ, Hunsicker LG, Clarke WR, et al. Renoprotective effects of the ARB irbesartan in patients with nephropathy due to type 2 diabetes (IDNT). N Engl J Med 2001;345:851–860.
104. Brenner BM, Cooper ME, deZeeuw D, et al. Effects of losartan on renal and CV outcomes in patients with type 2 diabetes in nephropathy. N Engl J Med 2001;345:861–869.
105. Dahlof B, Sever P, Poulter N, et al. Prevention of CV events with an antihypertensive regimen of amlodipine adding perindopril as required vs atenolol adding bendroflumethiazide as required. Lancet 2005;366:895–906.
106. Wild S, Lee A, Fowkes G. Ankle-brachial pressure index and metabolic syndrome are independent predictors of CVD mortality in the Edinburgh Artery Study Cohort. Circulation 2004;109(6):72.
107. Selvin E, Erlinger TD. Prevalence and risk factors for PAD results from the NHANES 1999–2000. Circulation 2004;109(6):43.

Chapter 7
The Metabolic Syndrome and Obesity in Children and Adolescents

PREVALENCE

The prevalence of the metabolic syndrome in United States adolescents was estimated in the third National Health and Nutrition Examination Survey (NHANES-III) from 1988 to 1994. Among 1960 children aged 12 years or older who fasted at least 8 hours, two thirds had at least one metabolic abnormality, and almost one in 10 had the metabolic syndrome. The ethnic/racial distribution was similar to that in adults. Mexican Americans, followed by non-Hispanic whites, had a greater prevalence of the metabolic syndrome as compared to non-Hispanic blacks [1]. Almost one third of the overweight/obese adolescents had the metabolic syndrome. Childhood obesity predicts the metabolic syndrome in adulthood [4]. It is thought that 1 million U.S. adolescents meet the ATP-III criteria for the metabolic syndrome. The prevalence of the metabolic syndrome in adolescents is 4% overall, but it is 30% to 50% in overweight children [5]. Weiss et al [5] found that each half-unit increase in body mass index (BMI) (converted to a Z-score) was associated with a 50% increased risk of the metabolic syndrome in overweight children and adolescents. The metabolic syndrome has an immediate clinical effect, as supported by the fact that these children have a reduced exercise capacity compared to obese and normal-weight controls [6]. In a high-risk population in the U.S., 39% children were found to have the metabolic syndrome when defined by BMI instead of waist circumference, lipid levels of >95th percentile (or <5th percentile for HDL), and oral glucose tolerance testing [5].

PATHOGENESIS

Q: What are the diagnostic criteria and pathogenesis of the metabolic syndrome in children and how does it affect the clinical management?

There is no standard pediatric definition of the metabolic syndrome. However, de Ferranti et al [1] defined the metabolic syndrome in adolescents and children (using Adult Treatment Panel [ATP-III] criteria) as three or more of the following criteria:

1. Fasting triglycerides ≥1.1 mmol/L (100 mg/L)
2. High-density lipoprotein (HDL) <1.3 mmol/L (50 mg/dL), except in boys aged 15 to 19 years: <1.2 mmol/L (45 mg/dL)
3. Fasting glucose ≥6.1 mmol/L (110 mg/dL)
4. Waist circumference ≥75th percentile for age and gender
5. Systolic blood pressure >90th percentile for gender, age, and height

Other definitions used slightly different criteria for the diagnosis of the metabolic syndrome, which affected the prevalence rates accordingly. The Quebec Family Cohort Study used skinfold measurements and mean blood pressure [2]. A Hungarian study used more extreme lipid cutoff points, body fat measurements instead of waist circumference, and 24-hour blood pressure monitoring. There is a strong association among insulin resistances, being overweight, abnormal lipids, and high blood pressure in childhood and adolescence.

Canadian researchers have generated, for the first time, criteria for the metabolic syndrome specific to adolescents; the criteria develop a growth curve model [3]. Age- and sex-specific cutoff points for each metabolic component, blood pressure, triglyceride, HDL cholesterol, and waist circumference were used to generate age-related growth curves, similar to the ones used routinely by pediatricians. Tables were also constructed as an alternative to the growth curves [3].

Q: How does the pathogenesis of the metabolic syndrome in childhood and adolescence differ from that in the adult?
The pathophysiology of the metabolic syndrome is essentially similar to that in adults. Some pediatric investigators studied individual metabolic abnormalities that increase the cardiovascular (CV) risk and noted that the abnormalities start from childhood and go into adulthood, leading to the notion that the metabolic syndrome also tracks into adulthood [5]. The metabolic syndrome is thought to be triggered by a combination of genetic factors and environmental factors, such as excess calorie intake, reduced physical activity, and smoking. The effects of dietary composition on insulin resistance, however, are poorly understood. Insulin resistance may develop before adulthood in high-risk individuals, such as in children with a parental history of insulin resistance syndrome. This is because the genetic and environmental factors

are shared within families. Twin and family studies have found substantial familial aggregation of the insulin resistance syndrome as well as for each of the components of the metabolic syndrome [7]. Thus, parental insulin resistance is a predictor of the insulin resistance syndrome in childhood, despite the absence in children of differences in the conventional insulin resistance syndrome criteria currently used for diagnosis in adults. By contrast, there were no differences in insulin resistance between children with and those without an obese parent, despite significant differences in adiposity between these children [7].

Excess Calorie Intake and Reduced Physical Activity

The primary cause of the metabolic syndrome is thought to be obesity and the resulting hyperinsulinemia, which is associated with elevated blood pressure and lipid abnormalities. As discussed previously, insulin resistance has multiple various effects such as excessive hepatic production of very low density lipoprotein (VLDL) cholesterol, the resistance of insulin action on lipoprotein lipase in peripheral tissues, increased cholesterol synthesis, increased HDL cholesterol degradation, increased sympathetic activity, proliferation of smooth muscle cells, and increased formation and decreased reduction of plaque [8]. The role of leptin, adiponectin, interleukin-6 (IL-6), tumor necrosis factor-α (TNF-α), and plasminogen activator inhibitor-1 (PAI-1) is more or less similar. A direct association between obesity and insulin resistance has also been seen in children, as has the association between insulin resistance and lipids [9]. Obesity in childhood and during adolescence is associated with high levels of fasting insulin, lipids, and blood pressure in young adulthood. Weight loss in these children can decrease insulin levels, and increase insulin sensitivity toward normal in adults and adolescence.

ASSESSMENT

It is important to identify the children who would benefit from intervention. Fasting plasma glucose should be tested in those (1) who are overweight; (2) have a family history of type 2 diabetes; (3) have a predisposition according to race/ethnicity (American Indian, African American, Hispanic, or Asian/Pacific Islander); and (4) have signs of insulin resistance or conditions associated with insulin resistance (e.g., acanthosis nigricans, hypertension, dyslipidemia, or polycystic ovary syndrome).

Insulin resistance per se is assessed by the euglycemic clamp, which is primarily used for research only. An alternative method of a reasonable assessment of hyperinsulinemia is provided by measuring fasting plasma insulin level, which may provide a reasonable clinical alternative for evaluating insulin resistance (range: normal, <15 mU/L; borderline high, 15 to 20 mU/L; high, >20 mU/L). Blood pressure at a young age is a predictor of blood pressure elevation during later years of life. Hence, advice at a very early age is beneficial in preventing hypertension in adulthood. At 3 years of age, formal recording of blood pressure should begin [9].

A thorough family history is essential to detect those patients who are at risk according to race/ethnicity or familial predisposition. A physical examination should include assessment of obesity, and detection of signs of acanthosis nigricans, subcutaneous fat deposits, and signs of endocrinal disease (e.g., polycystic ovary syndrome, Cushing syndrome). Measurement of blood pressure, fasting glucose, and lipids is necessary. Weight control, lifestyle modifications in childhood, and early detection of type 2 diabetes could change the incidence of the metabolic syndrome and improve the risk profile for cardiovascular disease (CVD) and type 2 diabetes [9].

Evidence that the Metabolic Syndrome Increases Cardiovascular Risk

Q: What is the predictive power of cardiovascular disease and type 2 diabetes in childhood metabolic syndrome?
The metabolic syndrome has a marked effect on CVD risk in the young. Steinberger et al [10] suggested that obesity in the young is associated with hyperinsulinemia, reduced insulin sensitivity, and increased total cholesterol and triglycerides [10]. An increase in body mass index (BMI) during childhood is considered to be the most important risk factor for the metabolic syndrome. However, in children, the relationship between the components of metabolic syndrome and its role as a predictor of adult CVD and type 2 diabetes is not entirely clear [9]. However, recent reports suggest an alarming increase in the incidence of type 2 diabetes in children.

CARDIOVASCULAR DISEASE
Pankow et al [7] found that the metabolism syndrome has a strong association with CVD risk factors. The Muscatine Study [11] and Bogalusa Study [12] have shown that obesity during childhood and adolescence is the cause of CV risk factors including dyslipidemia

(increased triglycerides, reduced HDL cholesterol), hypertension, left ventricular hypertrophy, obstructive sleep apnea, and atherosclerosis. There is sufficient evidence to show that obesity in childhood is positively related to elevated blood pressure. This is substantiated in both the Muscatine and Bogalusa studies, which have shown that increased BMI is consistently associated with high blood pressure. In the Muscatine study, adult blood pressure was shown to be related to the alteration in BMI from childhood to adulthood. Mahoney et al [13] followed the presence of coronary artery calcium in young adults who had already been studied as children in the Muscatine study. They found that in the age group 29 to 37 year old, the prevalence of coronary artery calcification was 31% in men and 10% in women. The important determinants of coronary artery calcium included weight in childhood, BMI in young adulthood, and BMI at the time of the study, with the odds ratio ranging from 3.0 to 6.1.

In adults, left ventricular hypertrophy is the known risk factor for CVD. Left ventricular hypertrophy has been shown to be associated with childhood obesity. Daniels et al [14] found that lean body mass, fat mass, and systolic blood pressure were independently associated with left ventricular mass in children and adults. Obstructive sleep apnea, an emerging CV risk factor, has been shown to be associated with obesity in children and adults. Amin et al [15] found that increased BMI in children was associated with increased risk of obstructive apnea, which in turn was associated with increased left ventricular mass index.

Bogalusa Study

Berenson et al [12] performed autopsies on 204 young persons, 2 to 39 years of age, who had died from accidental causes. Then they correlated the risk factors with the extent of atherosclerotic aortic and coronary arteries. Their study clearly showed a strong correlation between coronary atherosclerotic lesions and CV risk factors in the young. Their antemortem risk factors, such as elevated BMI, elevated systolic blood pressure, elevated low-density lipoprotein (LDL) cholesterol level, elevated triglyceride level, and cigarette smoking, are significantly related to the extent of atherosclerotic lesions in young people. There was a positive correlation between the extent of fatty streak and that of fibrous plaques, which was greater in the coronary arteries than in the aorta. Also, the proportion of collagenous fibrous plaques in relation to fatty streak was greater in the coronary vessels than in the aorta. The authors found that a higher BMI was associated with more extensive fatty streaks in the coronary arteries in 15- to 24-year-old boys and men and in 25- to 34-year-old men.

The effect of BMI was independent and could not be explained by other CVD risk factors. The presence of multiple risk factors including obesity was also shown to predispose to atherosclerosis.

Left Ventricular Hypertrophy
Severe left ventricular hypertrophy (LVH) and abnormal left ventricular geometry are relatively prevalent in young patients with essential hypertension. These findings suggest that these patients may be at risk of future CVD [16]. Excess body mass may contribute to the elevation of blood pressure and the development of severe LVH. Weight loss is an important lifestyle intervention in reducing severe LVH. The lean body mass and fat mass are both statistically significant correlates of left ventricular mass. Identifying children with multiple CVD risk factors is important as individuals with multiple risk factors have a substantially increased CVD risk compared with those a single factor, and that risk factor level tends to cluster in individuals. The association between inflammation and obesity in youth is emerging, and this will increase the medical complications of obesity such as CVD.

TYPE 2 DIABETES
The increased incidence of type 2 diabetes in the young is reflected by increases in the prevalence of individuals with the metabolic syndrome who are overweight. Presently, type 2 diabetes occurs in adolescence typically at a BMI >30, a cutoff point classified as obese even in adults. According to NHANES-III, the prevalence of type 2 diabetes in U.S. adolescents is 4.1 in 1000, more than twice the prevalence of type 1 diabetes (1.7 in 1000). This increases the risk of CVD in later years, but the exact projection is hard to give at this stage. However, if these adolescents are subject to the trends found in adults, they will suffer CV outcomes in the third or fourth decade of their life—a frightening thought!

OBESITY

Q: What are the risk factors of obesity in children and adolescents?

Prevalence
In the United States the prevalence of childhood obesity tripled between 1980 and 2001 [17] and almost doubled between 1985 and 1995. Increases in obesity have also been observed in other countries, such as Canada, the United Kingdom, China, Germany, France, and Finland. The highest rates of obesity in the U.S. have occurred among African-American and Latino youth. The trend is

particularly concerning, as being overweight during childhood and adolescence is associated with an increased risk of hypertension, dyslipidemia, type 2 diabetes, and early atherosclerotic lesions as well as an increased risk of obesity and obesity-related morbidities and mortalities in adulthood.

The BMI is a suitable method of measuring obesity in children. For children in the U.S., being overweight is defined using the Centers for Disease Control and Prevention (CDC) age- and sex-specific nomograms for BMI. A normal BMI ranges from greater than the fifth percentile up to the <85th percentile; a BMI 85th percentile up to the 95th percentile is considered at risk for being overweight [16]; and a BMI ≥ 95th percentile is considered overweight. At late adolescence, these percentile are almost the same as the adult definitions; the 95th percentile is a BMI of 30. Obesity, therefore, should be defined as a BMI ≥ 95th percentile in children and adolescents.

The American Heart Association (AHA) suggests that it is reasonable to use the 85th percentile to identify those who are mildly to moderately overweight and the 95th percentile for those who are more significantly overweight. It is essential to calculate BMI in children who are in the 75th percentile or higher for height and weight because they are at the greatest risk of obesity. As in adults, obesity is the consequence of an imbalance between energy intake and energy expenditure. Adipose tissue is involved in feedback regulation of energy balance by the production of peptide hormones and leptin and adiponectin. The absence of leptin results in massive obesity. Adiponectin secreted by adipose tissue enhances insulin sensitivity and is an antiinflammatory cytokines. Metabolism of the adrenal steroid in adipose tissue may provide a process for increased visceral adiposity.

Children whose BMI is in the 95th percentile or higher should undergo blood pressure measurements, lipid profile analysis, fasting insulin, and glucose measurements. They should be examined thoroughly to assess for pseudotumor cerebri, nighttime snoring, breathing difficulties, or daytime somnolence, which may indicate obstructive sleep apnea or obesity hypoventilation syndrome. They also should be assessed for slipped capital femoral epiphysis, polycystic ovary disease, Cushing syndrome, type 2 diabetes, hepatic steatosis, thyroid disorders, Blount's disease, and psychological disorders. They will benefit from counseling and advice on a healthy diet, which is almost similar to that for adults. One half of a healthy meal should be salad and vegetables, one fourth should be starch (potatoes, rice, etc.), and one fourth should be protein (meat, poultry, fish, soya, etc.). For younger children, the parents would be counseled instead. Even a weight loss of 5 to 10 lb can confer substantial benefits. Children with complications of obesity (e.g., hypertension, elevated lipids, insulin resistance, hepatic steatosis) should lose enough weight to correct the complications. Behavioral treatments with overweight children produce long-term benefits.

Relationship Between Childhood Obesity and Adult-Type Obesity

There is a direct positive relationship between birth weight and the BMI attained later in live [18]. Rapid weight gain during infancy is also related to obesity in childhood, potentially reflecting an interaction of genetic and postnatal environmental factors [19]. Additionally, lower birth weight for gestational age is also associated with central obesity and increased CV risk [20]. Other data suggest that an early rebound of the BMI is associated with an increased risk of higher BMI in adulthood. The BMI rebound occurs in a period usually between 4 and 7 years of age. A recent study found early rebound to be associated with glucose intolerance and diabetes in adults [21]. The BMI at the age of 7 or 8 years is thought to be a good predictor of obesity, as is the age at BMI rebound. Some studies found that breast-feeding is associated with a lower risk of obesity during childhood and adolescence. This concept is not universally agreed upon. Girls have a higher risk of becoming obese than boys during adolescence. If the onset of obesity occurs during childhood, the obesity is more likely to continue during later years of life. Obesity during adolescence is shown to be associated with an increased overall mortality and specifically with an increased risk of CVD and diabetes in adulthood [22].

Although dyslipidemia can be diagnosed in infancy, intervention is not usually required before 2 years of age. A reasonable age for this assessment is 2 to 6 years. On population studies, childhood cholesterol level is a good predictor of cholesterol level in young adulthood.

Drug therapy to lower the blood cholesterol level is reserved for those 10 years of age or older who, despite being on treatment, have an LDL cholesterol persistently ≥190 mg/dL (4.9 mmol/L) or an LDL cholesterol >160 mg/dL (4.2 mmol/L) and either a strong family history of premature coronary artery disease (CAD) or two or more adult CVD risk factors (e.g., low HDL cholesterol, smoking, high blood pressure, obesity, or diabetes). Because more than one fifth of U.S. adolescents smoke cigarettes on a daily basis by the time they are in high school, smoking cessation is advised. For infants and very young children, intervention is directed not at the child but at parents who smoke, because of the risk for children from passive smoking.

The dairy factors that are linked to insulin resistance syndrome include low dairy consumption, a low ratio of monosaturated or polysaturated to saturated fatty acids, a diet low in fiber, and a high glycemic index. High dairy consumption seems to have favorable effects on body weight in children and adults. In addition, high dairy and calcium consumption may decrease the risk for hypertension, coagulopathy, CAD, and stroke [9]. Dietary patterns characterized by increased consumption have an inverse association with insulin resistance syndrome among overweight adults and may reduce the risk of type 2 diabetes and CVD [23]. Diary products may have favorable effects on body weight in children and adults. The Coronary Artery Risk Development in Young Adults (CARDIA) study, a population-based prospective study, observed an inverse association between the frequency of diary intake and the development of obesity, abnormal glucose homeostasis, elevated blood pressure, and dyslipidemia in overweight black and white young men and women. The 10-year incidence of the metabolic syndrome was lower by more than two thirds among overweight individuals in the highest category of diary consumption ($\geq$ 5 servings/d) compared with those in the lowest category (<1.5 servings/d). These associations were not compounded by other lifestyle factors or dietary variables that are correlated with diary intake and did not differ materially by race or sex [23].

Although saturated fat contained in dairy products may raise the LDL cholesterol levels, there are several mechanisms by which diary intake may protect against insulin resistance, obesity, and CVD [23]. Some studies suggest that calcium, potassium, and magnesium may lower the risk of hypertension, CHD, stroke, and type 2 diabetes. It is also likely that the lactose protein and fat in dairy food may enhance satiety and reduce the risk of being overweight or obese relative to other high-carbohydrate foods and beverages. The low glycemic index associated with dairy products may also play role. The association between metabolic syndrome and dairy intake was not observed in individuals who were not overweight. Dairy products may thus protect against obesity and the metabolic syndrome.

Physical Activity

One study found a graded negative association between the clustering of risk factors and physical activity. It was recommended that the physical activity level should be higher than the current international guidelines of at least 1 hour per day of physical activity of at least moderate intensity to prevent a cluster of CVD risk factors [24].

References

1. de Ferranti S, Gauvreau K, Ludwig DS, et al. Prevalence of metabolic syndrome in American adolescents. Circulation 2004;110:2994–2997.

2. Katzmarzyk PT, Perusse L, Malina RM, et al. Stability of indicators of the metabolic syndrome from childhood and adolescence to young adulthood. J Clin Epidemiol 2001:54:190–195.

3. Jollife J, Janssen I. Development of age-specific adolescent metabolic syndrome criteria that are link to the ATPIII and IDF criteria. J Am Coll Cardiol 2007;49:891–898.

4. Vanhala MJ, Vanhala PT, Keinanen-Kiukaannieme SM, et al. Relative weight gain and obesity as a child predict metabolic syndrome as an adult. Int J Obes Relat Metab Disord 1999;23:656–659.

5. Weiss R, Dziura J, Burgert TS, et al. Obesity and the metabolic syndrome in children and adolescents. N Engl J Med 2004;350:2362–2374.

6. Torok K, Szelenyi Z, Porszasz J, et al. Low physical performance in obese adolescent boys with metabolic syndrome. Int J Obes Relat Metab Disord 2001;25:966–970.

7. Pankow JS, Jacobs DR Jr, Steinberger J, et al. Insulin resistance and cardiovascular disease risk factors in children of parents with the metabolic syndrome. Diabetes Care 2004;27:775–780.

8. Stephen R, Daniels MD, Donna K, et al. AHA scientific statement, overweight in children and adolescents. Circulation 2005;111:1999–2012.

9. Williams CL, Hayman LL, Daniels SR, et al. Cardiovascular health in childhood. Circulation 2002;106:143–160.

10. Steinberger J, Moran A, Hong CP, et al. Adiposity in childhood predicts obesity and insulin resistance in young adulthood. J Pediatr 2001;138:469–473.

11. Lauer RM, Lee J, Clarke WR. Factors affecting the relationship between childhood and adult cholesterol levels: the Muscatine Study. Pediatrics 1988;82:209–318.

12. Berenson GS, Srinivasan SR, Bao et al. Association between multiple CV risk factors and atherosclerosis is children & young adults. N. Engl J Med 1998;338:1650–1656.

13. Mahoney LT, Burns TL, Stanford W, et al. Coronary risk factors measured in childhood and young adult life is associated with coronary artery calcification in young adults: the Muscatine Study. J Am Coll Cardiol 1996;27:277–284.

14. Daniels SR, Kimball TR, Morrison JA, et al. Effect of lean body mass, fat mass, blood pressure, and sexual maturation on left ventricular mass in children and adolescents. Circulation 1995;92:3249–3254.

15. Amin RS, Kimball TR, Bean JA, et al. Left ventricular hypertrophy and abnormal ventricular geometry in children and adolescents with obstructive sleep apnea. Am J Respir Crit Care Med 2002;165:1395–1399.

16. Ogden CL, Flegae KM, Carroll MD, et al. Prevalence & trends in overweight among US children & adolesants. 1999–2000 JAMA 2002; 288;1728–1732.

17. Ogden CL, Kuczmarski RJ, Flegal KM et al. Centers for Disease Control and Prevention 2000 growth charts for the US. Pediatrics 2002;109:45–60.

18. Parsons TJ, Power C, Logan S, et al. Childhood predictors of adult obesity: a systematic review. Int J Obes Relat Metab Disord 1999;23:S1–S107.

19. Stettler N, Zemel BS, Kumanyika S, et al. Infant weight gain and childhood overweight status in a multicenter, cohort study. Pediatrics 2002;109:194–199.

20. Barker M, Robinson S, Osmond C, et al. Birth weight and body fat distribution in adolescent girls. Arch Dis Child 1997;77:381–383.

21. Bhargava SK, Sachdev AS, Fall CH, et al. Relation of serial changes in childhood body-mass index to impaired glucose tolerance in young adulthood. N Engl J Med 2004;350:865–875.

22. Must A. Does overweight in childhood have an impact on adult healthy? Nutr Rev 2003;61:139–142.

23. Perera M, Jacobs D, Van H, et al. Dairy consumption, obesity, and the insulin resistance in young adults: the CARDIA study. JAMA 2002; 287:2081–2089.

24. Anderson LB, Harro M, Sardinha L, et al. Physical activity and clustered CV risk in children. Lancet 2006;368:299–304.

Index

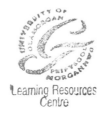

Learning Resources
Centre

Printed in the United States of America.